Diabetes and Cancer: Association, Mechanism, and Therapeutic Implications

Rana Noor
Editor

Diabetes and Cancer: Association, Mechanism, and Therapeutic Implications

Springer

Editor
Rana Noor
Department of Biochemistry
Jamia Millia Islamia
New Delhi, Delhi, India

ISBN 978-981-95-5650-2 ISBN 978-981-95-5651-9 (eBook)
https://doi.org/10.1007/978-981-95-5651-9

This Springer imprint is published by the registered company Springer Nature Singapore Pte Ltd.
The registered company address is: 152 Beach Road, #21-01/04 Gateway East, Singapore 189721, Singapore

Preface

Diabetes mellitus and cancer represent two of the most prevalent and complex noncommunicable diseases of the modern era, posing substantial challenges to global health systems. Increasing epidemiological and molecular evidence indicates that these disorders are not independent entities but are biologically interconnected through overlapping pathophysiological pathways. This convergence is driven by shared etiological factors such as obesity, sedentary lifestyle, aging, and nutritional imbalance, as well as by intrinsic cellular and molecular mechanisms involving chronic low-grade inflammation, oxidative stress, hyperinsulinemia, and insulin resistance. These factors collectively establish a systemic milieu that promotes both metabolic dysfunction and tumorigenesis.

From a mechanistic standpoint, persistent hyperglycemia and hyperinsulinemia facilitate abnormal cellular proliferation, angiogenesis, and inhibition of apoptosis, thereby enhancing oncogenic potential. In parallel, the pro-inflammatory and oxidative environment characteristic of diabetes contributes to DNA damage, mutagenesis, and immune evasion, the core hallmarks of cancer. Conversely, cancer therapies such as chemotherapy, radiotherapy, endocrine treatment, and emerging immunotherapeutic regimens can exacerbate metabolic disturbances by impairing pancreatic β-cell function, altering insulin signaling, and inducing glucocorticoid-mediated hyperglycemia. These reciprocal interactions underscore the bidirectional relationship between diabetes and cancer and highlight the necessity for integrated metabolic and oncologic management.

The accelerating incidence of both diseases necessitates a unified research framework to elucidate their molecular intersections and to develop preventive and therapeutic strategies that address their common biological roots. This book provides a comprehensive scientific synthesis of the mechanisms linking diabetes and cancer, integrating perspectives from molecular biology, endocrinology, oncology, and translational medicine. The contributing chapters collectively examine epidemiological correlations, mechanistic pathways, clinical implications, and emerging therapeutic paradigms that define this dual disease burden.

Through the consolidation of recent evidence and interdisciplinary analysis, this volume aims to advance understanding of the pathophysiological continuum between metabolic and neoplastic processes. It emphasizes the importance of early metabolic monitoring in oncology, presents pharmacological agents with dual antidiabetic and anticancer effects, and the design of preventive strategies rooted in precision medicine. The scientific insights presented herein are intended to foster translational research and guide the development of integrated healthcare models that can mitigate the global impact of these interrelated disorders.

New Delhi, Delhi, India Rana Noor

Contents

Editor and Contributors

About the Editor

Rana Noor is currently working as an Assistant Professor at Jamia Millia Islamia, New Delhi, with a PhD in Biochemistry from AMU (Aligarh Muslim University). She is an accomplished biochemist and educator with a rich academic and professional history. Her research interest spans areas such as papain inactivation, the effects of oxygen-derived free radicals, and the activation of CFTR (cystic fibrosis transmembrane conductance regulator) by genistein. She has published several research articles and is an editorial board member of numerous international and national journals. Her research contributions, recognized with Best Paper Awards and invitations to review for international conferences, attest to her exceptional expertise in the field.

Contributors

Ashiq Shibili P Medical Biotechnology Lab, Faculty of Allied Health Sciences, Chettinad Hospital and Research Institute (CHRI), Chettinad Academy of Research and Education (CARE), Chennai, TN, India

Antara Banerjee Medical Biotechnology Lab, Faculty of Allied Health Sciences, Chettinad Hospital and Research Institute (CHRI), Chettinad Academy of Research and Education (CARE), Chennai, TN, India

Praveen Kumar Chandra Sekar Human Cytogenetics and Genomics Laboratory, Faculty of Allied Health Sciences, Chettinad Hospital and Research Institute, Chettinad Academy of Research and Education, Kelambakkam, TN, India

Mamali Das Department of Biomedical Science, Faculty of Science, Alagappa University, Karaikudi, TN, India

Arumugam Kamaladevi Department of Biomedical Science, Faculty of Science, Alagappa University, Karaikudi, TN, India

Chandramohan Kiruthiga Department of Biomedical Science, Faculty of Science, Alagappa University, Karaikudi, TN, India

K. Langeswaran Department of Biomedical Science, Faculty of Science, Alagappa University, Karaikudi, TN, India

Yupa Min Department of Pathology, Faculty of Medicine, Quest International University, Ipoh, Malaysia

Uthamalingam Murali Deparment of Surgery, Manipal University College Malaysia, Melaka, Malaysia

Jethendra Kumar Muruganantham Human Cytogenetics and Genomics Laboratory, Faculty of Allied Health Sciences, Chettinad Hospital and Research Institute, Chettinad Academy of Research and Education, Kelambakkam, TN, India

R. Muthuvel Department of Biochemistry, Karuna Medical College and Hospital, Palakkad, Kerala, India

Sibin Nambidi Medical Biotechnology Lab, Faculty of Allied Health Sciences, Chettinad Hospital and Research Institute (CHRI), Chettinad Academy of Research and Education (CARE), Chennai, TN, India

Arunkumar Radhakrishnan Department of Pharmacology, Chettinad Hospital and Research Institute (CHRI), Chettinad Academy of Research and Education (CARE), Chennai, TN, India

Neeharika Sara Sennie Medical Biotechnology Lab, Faculty of Allied Health Sciences, Chettinad Hospital and Research Institute (CHRI), Chettinad Academy of Research and Education (CARE), Chennai, TN, India

Gowtham Kumar Subbaraj Faculty of Allied Health Science, Chettinad Hospital and Research Institute, Chettinad Academy of Research and Education, Kelambakkam, TN, India

Ramakrishnan Veerabathiran Human Cytogenetics and Genomics Laboratory, Faculty of Allied Health Sciences, Chettinad Hospital and Research Institute, Chettinad Academy of Research and Education, Kelambakkam, TN, India

An Overview of Diabetes and Cancer Risks: Types and Mechanisms

Jethendra Kumar Muruganantham and Ramakrishnan Veerabathiran

Abstract

Diabetes mellitus and cancer are major global health concerns, with growing evidence suggesting a strong interrelationship between the two. Epidemiological studies show that patients with diabetes, precisely type 2 diabetes, have an increased risk of acquiring numerous malignancies, such as pancreatic, liver, breast, colorectal, and endometrial cancer. The underlying mechanisms linking diabetes and cancer involve chronic hyperinsulinemia, insulin resistance, and systemic inflammation, which promote cellular proliferation and tumor progression. Metabolic dysregulation in diabetes alters various signaling pathways, such as IGF-1 and PI3K/AKT, facilitating oncogenesis. Certain antidiabetic medications influence cancer risk, with metformin showing potential anticancer properties, whereas insulin and sulfonylureas have been allied with an amplified risk of some cancers. Lifestyle factors, like obesity, poor dietary habits, and physical inactivity, contribute to both diabetes and cancer development, highlighting the importance of preventive strategies. Regular physical activity, a diet rich in fiber and antioxidants, and sidestepping smoking and alcohol can mitigate these risks. Pharmacological interventions, including personalized medicine approaches and genetic screening, may refine risk assessment and treatment strategies. The bidirectional relationship between diabetes and cancer underscores the need for comprehensive management strategies integrating metabolic and oncologic care. Early screening and timely interventions can improve patient outcomes. Despite the present understanding, gaps remain in identifying precise molecular mechanisms and practical therapeutic approaches. Further research should focus on

J. K. Muruganantham · R. Veerabathiran (✉)
Human Cytogenetics and Genomics Laboratory, Faculty of Allied Health Sciences, Chettinad Hospital and Research Institute, Chettinad Academy of Research and Education, Kelambakkam, Tamilnadu, India

R. Noor (ed.), *Diabetes and Cancer: Association, Mechanism, and Therapeutic Implications*, https://doi.org/10.1007/978-981-95-5651-9_1

developing targeted therapies that address the shared pathophysiology of diabetes and cancer. Increasing awareness among healthcare professionals and patients about the link between these conditions is essential for reducing disease burden and improving long-term prognosis.

Keywords

Diabetes · Cancer · Cellular mechanism · Medication · Prevention

1 Introduction

Diabetes mellitus (DM) is a chronic metabolic condition marked by high blood sugar levels caused by inadequate insulin synthesis, inefficient insulin usage, or both. This disorder severely influences the body's capacity to turn food into energy, leading to health complications if left unmanaged (Kitabchi et al., 2009). The most common types of diabetes are type 1 and type 2. Type 1 diabetes is an autoimmune illness in which the immune system targets insulin-producing beta cells in the pancreas, causing little or no insulin production (Yameny, 2024). Conversely, type 2 diabetes, which accounts for roughly 90–95% of diabetes cases worldwide, develops when the body becomes insulin-resistant or fails to generate enough insulin to maintain normal glucose levels (Alam et al., 2014).

The global burden of diabetes is staggering, with an estimated 830 million people affected as of 2022. This figure represents a significant increase from previous decades and highlights a rising public health calamity, predominantly in low- and middle-income countries (WHO, 2022). Diabetes is associated with numerous complications, including cardiovascular disease, kidney failure, and neuropathy, contributing to approximately 4.2 million deaths annually (Fan, 2017). Recent research has also explored the biological links between diabetes and cancer (Table 1).

Persons with diabetes are at a heightened risk for certain types of cancer, including pancreatic, liver, and colorectal cancers (Wang et al., 2020). The mechanisms underlying this association may involve insulin resistance and chronic inflammation, which can promote tumor development. Understanding these connections is vital for developing prevention strategies and improving outcomes for individuals with diabetes (Tsalamandris et al., 2019). One possible reason for the association

Table 1 Biological link between cancer and diabetes

Mechanism	Diabetes-associated changes	Cancer-promoting consequences
Metabolic dysregulation	High blood glucose levels	DNA damage, ROS production, alternative energy source for cancer cells
Hyperinsulinemia	Elevated insulin and IGF-1 levels	Promotes cell proliferation, differentiation, survival, metastasis
Chronic inflammation	Persistent inflammatory signals	Enhances tumor growth, EMT, immune evasion

between cancer and T2DM is the presence of common risk factors, such as obesity, smoking, and aging. Numerous malignancies, including those of the endometrium, breast, liver, pancreas, prostate, bladder, and colon, have been closely linked to type 2 diabetes (Giovannucci et al., 2010). The exact mechanisms connecting diabetes to cancer development remain unclear. However, several studies indicate potential contributing factors, including the insulin-like growth factor (IGF) pathway, elevated blood glucose levels, pro-inflammatory cytokines, and hormonal influences (Phua et al., 2018).

The intricate relationship between diabetes and cancer is increasingly evident, supported by epidemiological observations and biological insights. Shared risk factors such as obesity and aging, coupled with mechanisms like hyperinsulinemia, hyperglycemia, and chronic inflammation, subsidize the amplified cancer risk observed in diabetic individuals (Phua et al., 2018). Specifically, elevated insulin levels can promote cell proliferation, while high glucose levels and inflammation contribute to oxidative stress and tumorigenesis. Furthermore, genetic predispositions and processes like epithelial-to-mesenchymal transition (EMT) and endothelial-to-mesenchymal transition (EndMT) further intertwine diabetes and cancer development, emphasizing the need for comprehensive strategies addressing both conditions (Zhu & Qu, 2022).

The connection between diabetes and cancer is complex, driven by multiple interconnected mechanisms. Insulin resistance and the resulting hyperinsulinemia can enhance tumor growth by stimulating cell proliferation and inhibiting apoptosis by activating the PI3K/Akt/mTOR and MAPK/ERK signaling pathways (Zhang et al., 2024). Persistent hyperglycemia further contributes by intensifying the Warburg effect in cancer cells, promoting glycolysis and lactate production, thereby fostering a more aggressive cancer phenotype. Additionally, elevated glucose levels heighten oxidative stress and inflammation, exacerbating tumor progression. Obesity and metabolic dysfunction also play a crucial role, alongside genetic and epigenetic modifications that intertwine the pathogenesis of both conditions (García-Jiménez et al., 2016). These factors establish a tumor-promoting environment, underscoring the importance of integrative strategies targeting metabolic and inflammatory pathways in diabetes and cancer.

2 Cancer Types Commonly Associated with Diabetes

2.1 Pancreatic Cancer

People with diabetes have a heightened risk of developing various cancers, with powerful links to pancreatic, liver, colorectal, endometrial, and breast cancers. Additionally, diabetes has been associated with an increased incidence of bladder, stomach, and some rarer cancers. In the case of type 1 diabetes, a greater susceptibility to liver, pancreatic, kidney, esophageal, stomach, lung, thyroid, and squamous cell cancers, as well as leukemia, has been reported. Moreover, some research

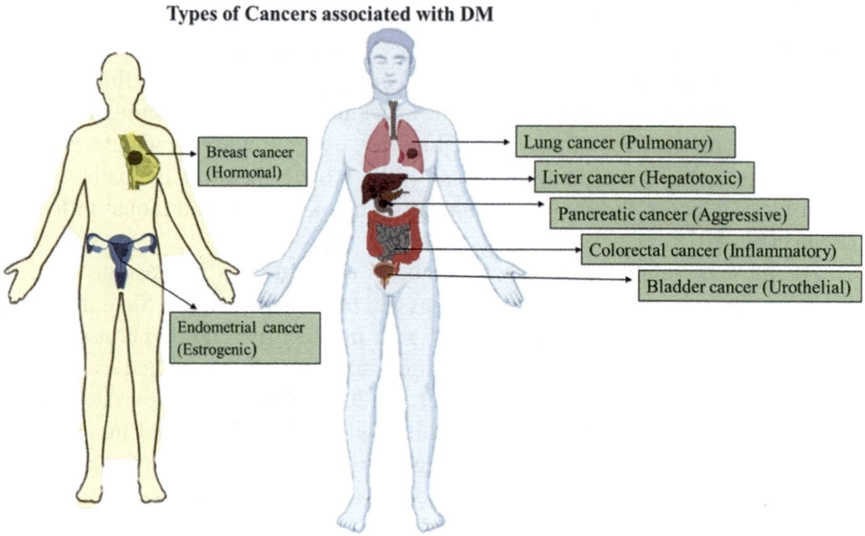

Fig. 1 Illustrates various types of cancers linked to diabetes, highlighting organ-specific cancer types such as breast cancer (hormonal), endometrial cancer (estrogenic), lung cancer (pulmonary), liver cancer (hepatotoxic), pancreatic cancer (aggressive), colorectal cancer (inflammatory), and bladder cancer (urothelial)

indicates that hyperglycemia may further elevate the risk of colorectal, liver, pancreatic, lung, and gastric cancers (Fig. 1) (Tsilidis et al., 2015).

Pancreatic cancer (PC) remains one of the deadliest cancers, with a 5-year survival rate of fewer than 10%. It is now the tenth most frequent cancer and the fourth major cause of cancer-related deaths in the USA. The connection between diabetes and PC has been recognized for nearly two centuries, with two main hypotheses emerging in recent research (Chaudhry et al., 2013). On the one hand, epidemiological studies indicate a significantly higher incidence of PC among individuals with diabetes, suggesting that diabetes may serve as a risk factor for PC. On the other hand, a potential early marker of PC, as the malignancy itself, can induce diabetes (Wang et al., 2020).

A bidirectional relationship between diabetes and PC was observed, with a time-dependent inverse risk pattern. The risk of developing PC is at its peak within the first 2 years after a diabetes diagnosis and gradually declines over time. In cases where diabetes persists for more than 5 years, the likelihood of PC becomes significantly lower (Muniraj & Chari, 2012). A 1.5- to twofold rise in the risk of PC has been allied with long-standing T2DM. PC development is influenced by insulin resistance, hyperglycemia, hyperinsulinemia, and chronic inflammation (Li, 2012). Cell proliferation is stimulated by insulin, creating a cycle that promotes cancer cell growth. Additionally, new-onset diabetes has been recognized as a potential early warning sign of undiagnosed PC, as pancreatic function may be impaired by tumors, leading to diabetes (Fig. 2). The contribution of pancreatic tumors to the onset of

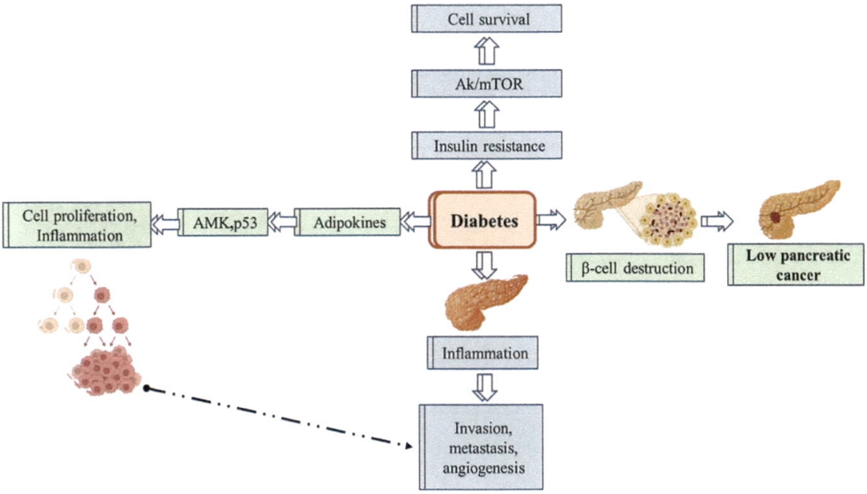

Fig. 2 Represents the mechanism of diabetes-induced pancreatic cancer and the biological pathways through which diabetes contributes to pancreatic cancer development. It depicts insulin resistance, β-cell destruction, chronic inflammation, and activation of signaling pathways like AMPK/p53 and AKT/mTOR that promote cell proliferation, survival, and metastasis

insulin resistance and diabetes has also been observed (Munigala et al., 2015). Consequently, it can be concluded that long-standing diabetes serves as a risk factor for PC, whereas new-onset diabetes acts as a potential indicator of the disease.

2.2 Liver Cancer (Hepatocellular Carcinoma)

People with T2DM have a two to four times higher chance of acquiring liver cancer (hepatocellular carcinoma) than people without the disease. This condition is a key risk factor for the disease (Mukherjee et al., 2015). This link is partially due to the liver's function in blood sugar management; when blood sugar levels remain high, extra fat accumulates, contributing to nonalcoholic fatty liver disease (NAFLD) growth. NAFLD can progress to nonalcoholic steatohepatitis (NASH), cirrhosis, and ultimately liver cancer (Onikanni et al., 2022). Insulin resistance, liver damage, higher pro-inflammatory cytokines, and even specific diabetic treatments have been linked to this development (Fig. 3).

In addition, hyperglycemia has been related to an amplified risk of distant metastasis in patients with hepatocellular carcinoma (Byrne & Targher, 2015). Lifestyle changes, including keeping a healthy weight, eating a balanced diet, and engaging in regular physical activity, can help control diabetes and minimize the risk of liver cancer (Chen et al., 2021). A prospective cohort study in Taiwan, a region with a high prevalence of hepatitis virus infections, investigated the association between diabetes and HCC. Among the 549,791 individuals screened, 5732 were diagnosed with diabetes and were followed until HCC was detected. The findings revealed that

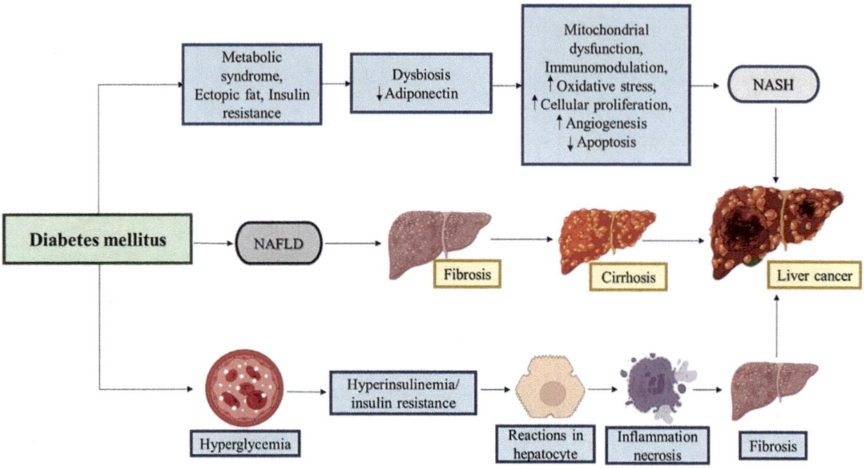

Fig. 3 Biological link between diabetes and liver cancer progression illustrates the role of diabetes mellitus in liver cancer progression through metabolic alterations, insulin resistance, hyperglycemia, inflammation, and liver conditions such as nonalcoholic fatty liver disease (NAFLD), fibrosis, cirrhosis, and hepatocellular carcinoma

individuals with diabetes who were HCV-negative had a complex risk of emerging HCC related to those who were HCV-positive (Lai et al., 2006). Additionally, NAFLD develops in over 70% of individuals with diabetes as a result of insulin resistance, increasing their susceptibility to severe liver conditions such as HCC (Mantovani & Targher, 2017). Several meta-analyses and systematic reviews have also identified NAFLD as a key factor linking diabetes to HCC (Wang et al., 2014).

2.3 Colorectal Cancer

The gut microbiota significantly influences colorectal cancer (CRC) growth and development. Unlike healthy individuals, CRC patients often exhibit dysbiosis, an imbalance in the gut microbiota. This imbalance leads to an increase in pro-carcinogenic bacteria, while beneficial commensal bacteria decrease. Specific bacteria, such as *Bacteroides fragilis, Escherichia coli, and Fusobacterium nucleatum,* have been closely linked to colorectal carcinogenesis (Kaviyarasan et al., 2024). These bacteria promote tumor development through various mechanisms, including triggering inflammatory responses, inducing DNA damage, and creating an immune environment favorable to tumor growth (Pandey et al., 2023). In contrast, CRC patients tend to have reduced levels of beneficial bacteria like *Roseburia.* Additionally, the gut microbiota may influence the effectiveness of immunotherapy and other CRC treatments (Kim & Lee, 2022).

While the dysregulation of the insulin pathway in colorectal cancer is not explicitly highlighted in the search results, it represents an important area of study connecting diabetes to colorectal cancer. Insulin resistance and hyperinsulinemia, common in type 2 diabetes, have been shown to activate the PI3K/Akt/mTOR and MAPK/ERK signaling pathways. These pathways, in turn, promote cell proliferation and inhibit apoptosis, processes linked to the onset and progression of various cancers, including colorectal cancer. As a result, individuals with diabetes may face a higher risk and more aggressive forms of colorectal cancer if the insulin pathway is disrupted (Yu et al., 2022). Notably, several studies have consistently demonstrated sex differences in diabetes risk, with males showing a significantly higher likelihood of developing the condition, while females exhibit a somewhat higher risk (Erbach et al., 2012) (Campbell et al., 2010). Even when both men and women follow a similarly healthy diet, research has shown that only women may experience a reduction in their risk of CRC. Diet plays a critical part in the progress of both diabetes and CRC (Wang et al., 2020).

2.4 Breast Cancer

Complex interactions between insulin and estrogens influence the growth of breast cancer. Insulin can enhance estrogen-dependent breast cancer by increasing estrogen production and bioactivity, stimulating sex steroid hormone receptor expression in tumor cells, and inducing aromatase activity in adipose stromal cells (Rose & Vona-Davis, 2012). Elevated insulin levels have been shown to promote cell proliferation in breast cancer cell lines and normal breast tissue. Studies propose that the heightened risk of breast cancer in women with high blood insulin levels, particularly in lean postmenopausal women, may be driven by mechanisms independent of obesity (Fig. 4).

Additionally, hyperinsulinemia may contribute to breast cancer risk by altering circulating estrogen levels. In both premenopausal and postmenopausal women, breast tumors are associated with increased estradiol levels (Gunter et al., 2009)

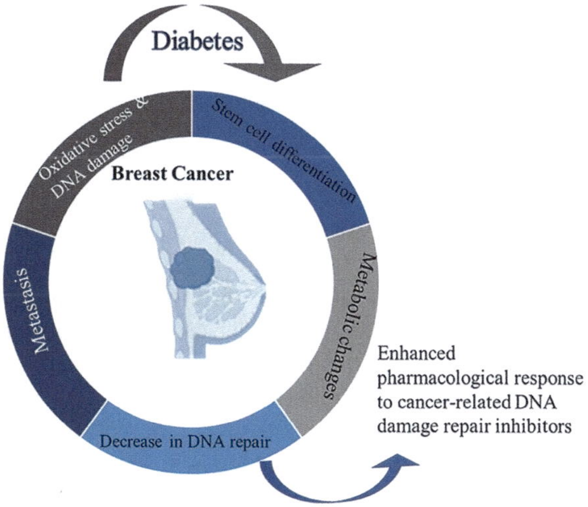

Fig. 4 Interrelationship between diabetes and cellular dysfunction, highlights the complex interactions between diabetes and key biological processes, including oxidative stress, DNA damage, and stem cell differentiation

(Mahmoud et al., 2019). The risk of breast cancer, particularly in postmenopausal women, can be elevated by factors such as increased circulating insulin due to insulin resistance, enhanced estrogen production in adipose tissue, and altered inflammatory markers, all of which are associated with obesity. Hyperinsulinemia, a result of insulin resistance, is more frequently observed in obese women (Catsburg et al., 2014). Additionally, the secretion of adipokines and cytokines produced by adipose tissue is influenced by obesity, with some promoting and others inhibiting carcinogenesis. These obesity-induced imbalances may create conditions that support breast cancer development. The risk of breast cancer can be lowered through regular physical exercise, a healthy diet, and successful weight control (Gunter et al., 2009). A study analyzed the influence of preexisting DM on BC outcomes. Women with diabetes exhibited a significantly higher overall mortality rate compared to those without the condition. Delivering radiation therapy to diabetic patients posed more significant challenges. Consequently, diabetes leads to postponed diagnosis and restricted treatment options, contributing to a more aggressive progression of BC and an elevated risk of mortality (Luo et al., 2015).

2.5 Endometrial Cancer

Endometrial cancer (EC) is primarily caused by hormonal imbalances and hyperglycemia, especially in those with diabetes mellitus (Byrne et al., 2020). As a separate risk factor, hyperglycemia, which is frequently seen in both T1 and T2DM, has been connected to an almost twofold higher occurrence of EC in women with DM than in those without the disease. Increased glycolysis and activating many signaling pathways are two ways a high-glucose environment promotes tumor development and invasiveness (Yang & Wang, 2019). Moreover, endometrial dysplasia and malignant transformation are influenced by diabetes-related hormonal changes, including increased insulin levels and impaired estrogen metabolism (Wang et al., 2022). The risk of cancer is further increased by endometrial cell proliferation, which is encouraged by insulin resistance and hyperinsulinemia. Therefore, reducing the incidence of EC and improving the prognosis for diabetic women require efficient blood glucose management and hormonal modulation (Mahema et al., 2024).

2.6 Bladder Cancer

The use of certain diabetes medications, including pioglitazone, has been linked with an amplified risk of bladder cancer. Pioglitazone, commonly prescribed for T2DM, may elevate this risk, particularly with prolonged use, as cautioned by the US Food and Drug Administration (FDA) (US FDA, 2016). A retrospective cohort study identified a significant association, reporting an adjusted hazard ratio of 1.63 for pioglitazone users compared to nonusers. Although some studies have presented conflicting evidence regarding this connection, the FDA advises caution when prescribing pioglitazone, especially for persons with a history of BC or those at high risk (US FDA, 2017). A meta-analysis of 36 observational studies indicated that while most investigations were conducted in Western countries, only one was conducted in Korea (Zhu et al., 2013).

The risk of bladder cancer may increase due to various diabetes-related alterations in the urinary system. Changes in urine composition and function caused by hyperglycemia and insulin resistance can lead to urinary tract infections and other complications (Lewis et al., 2011). These modifications may contribute to chronic inflammation and cellular damage in the bladder, creating a favorable environment for cancer development. Additionally, a higher prevalence of urinary symptoms and conditions, such as diabetic cystopathy, has been linked to diabetes, potentially worsening urinary health and further increasing cancer risk (MacKenzie et al., 2011).

2.7 Kidney Cancer

DM is recognized as an independent risk factor for kidney cancer, particularly renal cell carcinoma (RCC). Studies indicate that individuals with diabetes have a significantly higher likelihood of developing kidney cancer, with the risk being more pronounced in women and in certain regions, such as Asia (Bonilla-Sanchez et al., 2022). This association is primarily driven by hyperglycemia, hyperinsulinemia, and inflammatory processes that promote oxidative stress and uncontrolled cell proliferation. Additionally, diabetic patients diagnosed with kidney cancer often present with more aggressive disease characteristics, including a higher likelihood of recurrence and reduced overall survival rates. Furthermore, managing kidney cancer in diabetic patients can be more challenging, leading to poorer treatment outcomes compared to nondiabetic individuals (Labochka et al., 2016).

2.8 Lung Cancer

The link between diabetes and lung cancer is becoming increasingly important to understand. Recent research indicates that diabetes elevates the risk of developing lung cancer, particularly among smokers (Zhu & Qu, 2022). Insulin resistance and the chronic inflammation associated with diabetes are significant factors promoting lung tissue tumor growth. Although findings are not yet consistent, certain diabetes medications also have a potential impact on lung cancer risk. Furthermore, biological mechanisms such as metabolic dysregulation and alterations in immune responses create conditions that favor cancer development (Park et al., 2019). Further research must be conducted to clarify these associations definitively and to uncover the underlying pathways that connect DM with a heightened risk of lung cancer.

3 Role of Antidiabetic Medications in Cancer Risk

Insulin and Its Substitutes: An amplified risk of cancer has been linked with the use of insulin and its analogs, particularly combinations of intermediate- or long-acting and fast-acting insulin. Studies point to a possible link between insulin treatment and an increased risk of pancreatic and liver malignancies (Liu et al., 2019). More research is necessary to determine the precise processes behind this link.

3.1 Metformin

Several studies suggest that metformin may have a protective effect against liver and colorectal cancers. Research has shown that diabetic individuals taking metformin have up to a 62% lower risk of developing pancreatic cancer. Additionally, some studies indicate that metformin use may reduce the likelihood of liver cancer. However, conflicting evidence exists, as other studies have found no significant association between metformin use and cancer risk (Lee et al., 2018). Further research is necessary to clarify its role in cancer prevention.

3.2 Thiazolidinediones

Thiazolidinediones, including pioglitazone, have been related to a condensed risk of breast, lung, and liver cancers in certain studies. However, concerns have been raised regarding pioglitazone's potential to elevate the risk of bladder cancer, especially with long-term use. Due to this association, the FDA has issued warnings advising caution when prescribing pioglitazone, particularly for individuals at higher risk of bladder cancer (Chen et al., 2023).

3.3 Newer Medications (GLP-1 Agonists and SGLT2 Inhibitors)

Research suggests that dipeptidyl peptidase-4 (DPP-4) inhibitors may be related to a reduced risk of pancreatic cancer. However, the available data do not provide sufficient evidence to determine the cancer risk associated with glucagon-like peptide-1 (GLP-1) agonists and sodium-glucose co-transporter-2 (SGLT2) inhibitors (Garczorz et al., 2024). Further studies are needed to clarify their potential impact on cancer development.

4 Strategies for Screening and Prevention

Regular cancer screenings should be a fundamental aspect of routine healthcare for individuals with DM. Studies have shown that diabetes increases the risk of various cancers, with hepatocellular, pancreatic, breast, endometrial, and colorectal cancers.

Despite this heightened risk, cancer screening rates among diabetic patients remain significantly lower compared to nondiabetic individuals (Suh & Kim, 2019). To improve outcomes, screening recommendations should be tailored based on age and sex, with a strong emphasis on early detection. Recent advancements focus on developing blood tests capable of identifying individuals with newly diagnosed diabetes who may have a higher susceptibility to pancreatic cancer, allowing for earlier intervention and better disease management (Deligiorgi & Trafalis, 2023).

4.1 Changes in Lifestyle

Making lifestyle adjustments is vital for controlling diabetes and reducing cancer risk. A balanced diet rich in vegetables, fruits, whole grains, and fiber can help control blood sugar levels and promote general health. It is equally vital to be physically active regularly. To improve insulin sensitivity and help with weight control, aim for at least 150 minutes of reasonable exercise each week. It is also advised to limit alcohol intake because too much of it might harm cells and increase the chance of cancer (Hong, 2023).

4.2 Controlling Diabetes to Lower Cancer Risk

Proper diabetes management is crucial in reducing cancer risk. By regulating blood glucose levels through a mixture of diet, exercise, and medication, the molecular pathways that connect diabetes to cancer—such as hyperglycemia and chronic inflammation, can be mitigated. Effective diabetes control and regular monitoring enhance overall quality of life and significantly reduce the likelihood of developing diabetes-related cancers (Suh & Kim, 2019).

4.3 Ongoing Clinical Trials on Diabetes and Cancer

Numerous clinical trials are presently exploring the connection between diabetes and cancer, focusing on the effectiveness of various treatments and preventive strategies. These studies aim to assess the impact of different antidiabetic medications, such as GLP-1 agonists and metformin, on cancer outcomes. Additionally, researchers are investigating how glycemic control influences cancer incidence and progression, with some trials examining whether stricter glucose management may help lower cancer risk in individuals with diabetes (De Beer & Liebenberg, 2014).

4.4 Biomarkers for Cancer Risk in Diabetic Patients

Identifying biomarkers that can predict cancer risk in individuals with diabetes is an emerging field of research. Recent studies highlight the potential role of markers such as lactate dehydrogenase (LDH), C-reactive protein (CRP), and carcinoembryonic antigen (CEA) in assessing cancer susceptibility among diabetic patients. Elevated levels of these biomarkers have been associated with a higher incidence of cancer, suggesting their utility in early cancer detection and monitoring within this high-risk population. Additionally, research indicates that even prediabetic levels of glycated hemoglobin (HbA1c) may be connected to an augmented risk of cancer, underscoring the significance of metabolic markers in cancer risk assessment (Stan et al., 2023).

4.5 Methods of Personalized Medicine

Personalized medicine approaches, which tailor prevention and treatment strategies to an individual's unique biological profile, may be key to mitigating diabetes-related cancer risk in the future. When designing treatment plans, this method involves considering metabolic factors, genetic predispositions, and specific cancer types. Advances in proteomics and genomics could enable healthcare professionals to identify diabetic individuals at higher risk for certain cancers, more precisely facilitating targeted interventions (Table 2). Additionally, integrating pharmacological treatments with lifestyle modifications may enhance overall outcomes for diabetic patients at risk of cancer, promoting a comprehensive approach that addresses both metabolic and oncological health (Shahid et al., 2021).

Table 2 Biomarkers and personalized medicine for cancer risk in diabetic patients

Category	Biomarkers/factors	Relevance in cancer risk
Biomarkers for cancer risk	Lactate dehydrogenase (LDH)	Elevated levels linked to increased cancer incidence in diabetes
	C-reactive protein (CRP)	Indicates chronic inflammation, a known cancer risk factor
	Carcinoembryonic antigen (CEA)	Used for early cancer detection and monitoring
	Glycated hemoglobin (HbA1c)	High levels associated with increased cancer susceptibility
Personalized medicine approaches	Genetic profiling	Identifies individuals with a higher genetic predisposition
	Proteomics and genomics	Helps in targeted risk assessment and intervention strategies
	Pharmacological treatment	Integrates diabetes and cancer prevention therapies
	Lifestyle modifications	Enhances overall metabolic and oncological health

5 Conclusion

The interplay between diabetes mellitus and cancer is a complex and significant public health concern. Epidemiological and mechanistic studies indicate that diabetes, particularly type 2 diabetes, increases the risk of various cancers through metabolic dysregulation, chronic inflammation, and hormonal imbalances. Insulin resistance, hyperglycemia, and obesity contribute to tumor initiation and progression by activating oncogenic pathways. The impact of antidiabetic medications on cancer risk further complicates disease management, emphasizing the need for personalized treatment approaches. Given the overlapping risk factors, lifestyle modifications like maintaining a healthy weight, regular physical activity, and a stable diet play a vital part in dropping the incidence of both conditions. Early screening, genetic risk assessment, and integrated healthcare strategies can also enhance patient outcomes. However, gaps remain in understanding the precise molecular mechanisms linking diabetes and cancer, necessitating further research to develop targeted therapies. A multidisciplinary approach involving endocrinologists, oncologists, and researchers is essential to addressing this growing health challenge. By fostering awareness and advancing research, we can improve prevention, diagnosis, and treatment strategies, ultimately reducing the burden of diabetes and cancer globally.

Acknowledgement Thanks to the Chettinad Academy of Research and Education for their continuous support and encouragement.

References

Alam, U., Asghar, O., Azmi, S., & Malik, R. A. (2014). General aspects of diabetes mellitus. *Handbook of Clinical Neurology, 126*, 211–222.

Bonilla-Sanchez, A., Rojas-Munoz, J., & Garcia-Perdomo, H. A. (2022). Association between diabetes and the risk of kidney cancer: Systematic review and meta-analysis. *Clinical Diabetes, 40*(3), 270–282.

Byrne, C. D., & Targher, G. (2015). NAFLD: A multisystem disease. *Journal of Hepatology, 62*(1 Suppl), S47–S64.

Byrne, F. L., Martin, A. R., Kosasih, M., Caruana, B. T., & Farrell, R. (2020). The role of hyperglycemia in endometrial cancer pathogenesis. *Cancers (Basel), 12*(5), 1191.

Campbell, P. T., Deka, A., Jacobs, E. J., et al. (2010). Prospective study reveals associations between colorectal cancer and type 2 diabetes mellitus or insulin use in men. *Gastroenterology, 139*(4), 1138–1146.

Catsburg, C., Gunter, M. J., Chen, C., et al. (2014). Insulin, estrogen, inflammatory markers, and risk of benign proliferative breast disease. *Cancer Research, 74*(12), 3248–3258.

Chaudhry, Z. W., Hall, E., Kalyani, R. R., Cosgrove, D. P., & Yeh, H. C. (2013). Diabetes and pancreatic cancer. *Current Problems in Cancer, 37*(5), 287–292.

Chen, J. H., ATH, W., Lawal, B., et al. (2021). Identification of cancer hub gene signatures associated with immune-suppressive tumor microenvironment and ovatodiolide as a potential cancer immunotherapeutic agent. *Cancers (Basel), 13*(15), 384.

Chen, Y., Mushashi, F., Son, S., Bhatti, P., Dummer, T., & Murphy, R. A. (2023). Diabetes medications and cancer risk associations: A systematic review and meta-analysis of evidence over the past 10 years. *Scientific Reports, 13*(1), 11844.

de Beer, J. C., & Liebenberg, L. (2014). Does cancer risk increase with HbA1c, independent of diabetes? *British Journal of Cancer, 110*(9), 2361–2368.

Deligiorgi, M. V., & Trafalis, D. T. (2023). A concerted vision to advance the knowledge of diabetes mellitus related to immune checkpoint inhibitors. *International Journal of Molecular Sciences, 24*(8), 7630.

Erbach, M., Mehnert, H., & Schnell, O. (2012). Diabetes and the risk for colorectal cancer. *Journal of Diabetes and its Complications, 26*(1), 50–55.

Fan, W. (2017). Epidemiology in diabetes mellitus and cardiovascular disease. *Cardiovascular Endocrinology & Metabolism, 6*(1), 8–16. Published 2017 Feb 15.

García-Jiménez, C., Gutiérrez-Salmerón, M., Chocarro-Calvo, A., García-Martinez, J. M., Castaño, A., & De la Vieja, A. (2016). From obesity to diabetes and cancer: Epidemiological links and role of therapies. *British Journal of Cancer, 114*(7), 716–722.

Garczorz, W., Kosowska, A., & Francuz, T. (2024). Antidiabetic drugs in breast cancer patients. *Cancers, 16*(2), 299. Published 2024 Jan 10.

Giovannucci, E., Harlan, D. M., Archer, M. C., et al. (2010). Diabetes and cancer: A consensus report. *CA: a Cancer Journal for Clinicians, 60*(4), 207–221.

Gunter, M. J., Hoover, D. R., Yu, H., et al. (2009). Insulin, insulin-like growth factor-I, and risk of breast cancer in postmenopausal women. *Journal of the National Cancer Institute, 101*(1), 48–60.

Hong, J. W. (2023). Diabetes mellitus and cancer. *Cardiovascular Prevention and Pharmacotherapy, 5*(3), 69–73.

Kaviyarasan, V., Das, A., Deka, D., et al. (2024). Advancements in immunotherapy for colorectal cancer treatment: A comprehensive review of strategies, challenges, and future prospective. *International Journal of Colorectal Disease, 40*(1), 1.

Kim, J., & Lee, H. K. (2022). Potential role of the gut microbiome in colorectal cancer progression. *Frontiers in Immunology, 12*, 807648. Published 2022 Jan 7.

Kitabchi, A. E., Umpierrez, G. E., Miles, J. M., & Fisher, J. N. (2009). Hyperglycemic crises in adult patients with diabetes. *Diabetes Care, 32*(7), 1335–1343.

Labochka, D., Moszczuk, B., Kukwa, W., Szczylik, C., & Czarnecka, A. M. (2016). Mechanisms through which diabetes mellitus influences renal cell carcinoma development and treatment: A review of the literature. *International Journal of Molecular Medicine, 38*(6), 1887–1894.

Lai, M. S., Hsieh, M. S., Chiu, Y. H., & Chen, T. H. (2006). Type 2 diabetes and hepatocellular carcinoma: A cohort study in high prevalence area of hepatitis virus infection. *Hepatology, 43*(6), 1295–1302.

Lee, D. Y., Yu, J. H., Park, S., et al. (2018). The influence of diabetes and antidiabetic medications on the risk of pancreatic cancer: A nationwide population-based study in Korea. *Scientific Reports, 8*(1), 9719.

Lewis, J. D., Ferrara, A., Peng, T., et al. (2011). Risk of bladder cancer among diabetic patients treated with pioglitazone: Interim report of a longitudinal cohort study. *Diabetes Care, 34*(4), 916–922.

Li, D. (2012). Diabetes and pancreatic cancer. *Molecular Carcinogenesis, 51*(1), 64–74.

Liu, Y. C., Nguyen, P. A., Humayun, A., et al. (2019). Does long-term use of antidiabetic drugs changes cancer risk? *Medicine (Baltimore), 98*(40), e17461.

Luo, J., Hendryx, M., Virnig, B., et al. (2015). Pre-existing diabetes and breast cancer prognosis among elderly women. *British Journal of Cancer, 113*(5), 827–832.

MacKenzie, T., Zens, M. S., Ferrara, A., Schned, A., & Karagas, M. R. (2011). Diabetes and risk of bladder cancer: Evidence from a case-control study in New England. *Cancer, 117*(7), 1552–1556.

Mahema, S., Roshni, J., Raman, J., Ahmad, S. F., Al-Mazroua, H. A., & Ahmed, S. S. S. J. (2024). Molecular regulator driving endometriosis towards endometrial cancer: A multi-scale

computational investigation to repurpose anti-cancer drugs. *Cell Biochemistry and Biophysics, 82*(4), 3367–3381.
Mahmoud, A. S., Ali, N. I., Abuhadi, N. H., Atta, B. E., Abdalla, O. M., Hassan, A. M., Almohiy, H. M., Alasmari, N. M., & Bakheit, K. H. (2019). Estrogens, insulin status and interrelated lifestyle factors on females with breast carcinomas. *Onkologia i Radioterapia, 1*(4).
Mantovani, A., & Targher, G. (2017). Type 2 diabetes mellitus and risk of hepatocellular carcinoma: Spotlight on nonalcoholic fatty liver disease. *Annals of Translational Medicine, 5*(13), 270.
Mukherjee, B., Bhattacharya, S., Chakraborty, S., Satapathy, B. S., Dey, N. S., & Shaw, T. K. (2015). Is type 2 diabetes mellitus a predisposal cause for developing hepatocellular carcinoma? *Current Diabetes Reviews, 11*(2), 64–70.
Munigala, S., Singh, A., Gelrud, A., & Agarwal, B. (2015). Predictors for pancreatic cancer diagnosis following new-onset diabetes mellitus. *Clinical and Translational Gastroenterology, 6*(10), e118. Published 2015 Oct 22.
Muniraj, T., & Chari, S. T. (2012). Diabetes and pancreatic cancer. *Minerva Gastroenterologica e Dietologica, 58*(4), 331–345.
Onikanni, S. A., Lawal, B., Bakare, O. S., et al. (2022). Cancer of the liver and its relationship with diabetes mellitus. *Technology in Cancer Research & Treatment, 21*, 15330338221119743.
Pandey, H., Tang, D. W. T., Wong, S. H., & Lal, D. (2023). Gut microbiota in colorectal cancer: Biological role and therapeutic opportunities. *Cancers (Basel), 15*(3), 866.
Park, H. J., Joh, H. K., Choi, S., & Park, S. M. (2019). Type 2 diabetes mellitus does not increase the risk of lung cancer among never-smokers: A nationwide cohort study. *Translational Lung Cancer Research, 8*(6), 1073–1077.
Phua, W. W. T., Wong, M. X. Y., Liao, Z., & Tan, N. S. (2018). An aPPARent functional consequence in skeletal muscle physiology via peroxisome proliferator-activated receptors. *International Journal of Molecular Sciences, 19*(5), 1425.
Rose, D. P., & Vona-Davis, L. (2012). The cellular and molecular mechanisms by which insulin influences breast cancer risk and progression. *Endocrine-Related Cancer, 19*(6), R225–R241.
Shahid, R. K., Ahmed, S., Le, D., & Yadav, S. (2021). Diabetes and cancer: Risk, challenges, management and outcomes. *Cancers (Basel), 13*(22), 5735.
Stan, M. C., Georgescu, D., Mireştean, C. C., & Bădulescu, F. (2023). Cancer and diabetes: Predictive factors in patients with metabolic syndrome. *Diagnostics (Basel)., 13*(16), 2647.
Suh, S., & Kim, K. W. (2019). Diabetes and cancer: Cancer should be screened in routine diabetes assessment. *Diabetes and Metabolism Journal, 43*(6), 733–743.
Tsalamandris, S., Antonopoulos, A. S., Oikonomou, E., et al. (2019). The role of inflammation in diabetes: Current concepts and future perspectives. *European Cardiology Review, 14*(1), 50–59.
Tsilidis, K. K., Kasimis, J. C., Lopez, D. S., Ntzani, E. E., & Ioannidis, J. P. (2015). Type 2 diabetes and cancer: Umbrella review of meta-analyses of observational studies. *BMJ (Clinical research ed.), 350*, g7607.
US Food and Drug Administration. (2016). *FDA Drug Safety Communication: Updated FDA review concludes that the use of type 2 diabetes medicine pioglitazone may be linked to an increased risk of bladder cancer*. Available at http://www.fda.gov/Drugs/DrugSafety/ucm519616.htm. Accessed 27 Dec 2016.
US Food and Drug Administration. (2017). *Updated FDA review concludes that use of type 2 diabetes medicine pioglitazone may be linked to an increased risk of bladder cancer [Internet]*.
Wang, Y. G., Wang, P., Wang, B., Fu, Z. J., Zhao, W. J., & Yan, S. L. (2014). Diabetes mellitus and poorer prognosis in hepatocellular carcinoma: A systematic review and meta-analysis. *PLoS One, 9*(5), e95485.
Wang, M., Yang, Y., & Liao, Z. (2020). Diabetes and cancer: Epidemiological and biological links. *World Journal of Diabetes, 11*(6), 227–238.
Wang, Y., Zeng, X., Tan, J., Xu, Y., & Yi, C. (2022). Diabetes mellitus and endometrial carcinoma: Risk factors and etiological links. *Medicine (Baltimore), 101*(34), e30299.
World Health Organization. (2022). *Invisible numbers: The true extent of noncommunicable diseases and what to do about them*. World Health Organization.

Yameny, A. A. (2024). Diabetes mellitus overview 2024. *Journal of Bioscience and Applied Research, 10*(3), 641–645.

Yang, X., & Wang, J. (2019). The role of metabolic syndrome in endometrial cancer: A review. *Frontiers in Oncology, 9*, 744. Published 2019 Aug 8.

Yu, G. H., Li, S. F., Wei, R., & Jiang, Z. (2022). Colorectal cancer risk: Clinical and therapeutic implications. *Journal Diabetes Research, 2022*, 1747326.

Zhang, Y. Y., Li, Y. J., Xue, C. D., Li, S., Gao, Z. N., & Qin, K. R. (2024). Effects of T2DM on cancer progression: Pivotal precipitating factors and underlying mechanisms. *Frontiers in Endocrinology (Lausanne), 15*, 1396022.

Zhu, B., & Qu, S. (2022). The relationship between diabetes mellitus and cancers and its underlying mechanisms. *Frontiers in Endocrinology (Lausanne), 13*, 800995.

Zhu, Z., Wang, X., Shen, Z., Lu, Y., Zhong, S., & Xu, C. (2013). Risk of bladder cancer in patients with diabetes mellitus: An updated meta-analysis of 36 observational studies. *BMC Cancer, 13*, 310.

Understanding the Connection Between Diabetes and Cancer

Praveen Kumar Chandra Sekar
and Ramakrishnan Veerabathiran

Abstract

Diabetes and cancer are common chronic diseases worldwide, and emerging evidence highlights a strong connection between them. Epidemiological studies have suggested a link between diabetes mellitus and certain types of cancer. The risk of developing various forms of diabetes appears to increase in individuals with cancer. Conversely, some cancers and their treatment may lead to the onset of diabetes mellitus. Several factors contribute to the relationship between diabetes and cancer, including genetic predisposition, obesity, inflammation, hyperglycemia, cancer therapies, insulin levels, oxidative stress, and certain oral hypoglycemic medications. Understanding the complex interplay between these diseases is necessary to develop targeted prevention and treatment strategies. This chapter discusses the metabolic connections between cancer and diabetes and outlines the underlying mechanisms involved. It concludes by emphasizing the importance of an integrated, multidisciplinary approach to managing patients with both diabetes and cancer to improve overall patient outcomes.

Keywords

Diabetes mellitus · Cancer risk · Chronic inflammation · Oxidative stress · Obesity

---

P. K. Chandra Sekar · R. Veerabathiran (✉)
Human Cytogenetics and Genomics Laboratory, Faculty of Allied Health Sciences, Chettinad Hospital and Research Institute, Chettinad Academy of Research and Education, Kelambakkam, Tamil Nadu, India

R. Noor (ed.), *Diabetes and Cancer: Association, Mechanism, and Therapeutic Implications*, https://doi.org/10.1007/978-981-95-5651-9_2

1 Introduction

Diabetes and cancer are among the most pressing global health concerns, posing a significant burden on individuals and healthcare systems. Understanding the intricate relationship between these two chronic conditions is necessary to develop efficient prevention and treatment strategies. Diabetes has emerged as a significant global health challenge, affecting over 529 million people worldwide as of 2021, with projections suggesting that this number could rise to 1.3 billion by 2050 (Ong et al., 2023). Chronic high blood glucose levels characterize the disease due to defects in insulin production or action, primarily manifesting in two forms: Type 1 diabetes (T1D) and type 2 diabetes (T2D) are two primary forms of diabetes, with T2D accounting for approximately 95% of all cases and being closely associated with obesity, sedentary lifestyles, and dietary factors (American Diabetes Association, 2009). The rising prevalence of diabetes is concerning because it increases the risk of cardiovascular diseases and cancer (Matheus et al., 2013). Cancer remains a significant cause of mortality worldwide, with approximately 19.3 million new cases identified in 2020 (Sung et al., 2021). The complexity of cancer lies in its numerous types and subtypes, each of which has distinct risk factors and biological mechanisms. Table 1 represents the common risk factors linking diabetes and cancer.

Commonly diagnosed cancers include breast, lung, and colorectal cancers, of which lung cancer remains the most lethal (Dela Cruz et al., 2011). Shared risk factors for diabetes, such as obesity and chronic inflammation, further exacerbate the burden of cancer. As the prevalence of both diseases continues to increase, understanding their interrelationship becomes increasingly critical. Emerging research highlights a significant association between diabetes and various forms of cancer (Safadi et al., 2024). Individuals with diabetes are at an elevated risk of developing different forms of cancer, particularly endometrial, pancreatic, and liver cancers (Y. Wang et al., 2022). Some studies suggest that this increased risk is not solely attributable to shared factors such as obesity; instead, complex biological

Table 1 Common risk factors linking diabetes and cancer

Risk factor	Impact on diabetes	Impact on cancer
Obesity	Increases insulin resistance and chronic inflammation, leading to hyperglycemia	Obesity-induced inflammation promotes tumor growth
Chronic inflammation	Elevated levels of proinflammatory cytokines	Inflammatory cytokines drive cancer cell proliferation
Hyperglycemia	Excess blood glucose leads to oxidative stress	Fuels tumor growth by promoting angiogenesis
Sedentary lifestyle	Obesity, worsening metabolic control	Reduces immune function
Diet	Aggravates insulin resistance	Poor diet increases cancer risk by promoting inflammation
Smoking and alcohol	Induces insulin resistance	Risk factor for lung, liver, and pancreatic cancers

mechanisms are at play. Hyperglycemia, hyperinsulinemia, and chronic inflammation are believed to contribute to tumorigenesis in patients (Gallagher & LeRoith, 2015). Figure 1 illustrates the interplay of risk factors between diabetes and cancer.

Additionally, specific cancer treatments may induce or exacerbate diabetes, creating a cyclical relationship that complicates patient management (Shahid et al., 2021). This chapter aims to elucidate the connection between diabetes and cancer by exploring epidemiological evidence linking these two conditions. We will examine the underlying biological mechanisms of this association and discuss how shared risk factors contribute to increased cancer incidence among patients with diabetes. Furthermore, this chapter reviews present treatment protocols for managing patients with both diabetes and cancer, emphasizing the need for integrated care approaches that address both conditions simultaneously. The relationship between diabetes and cancer is thoroughly examined in this chapter, highlighting the need for early identification and specialized preventative measures for those who are at risk of both

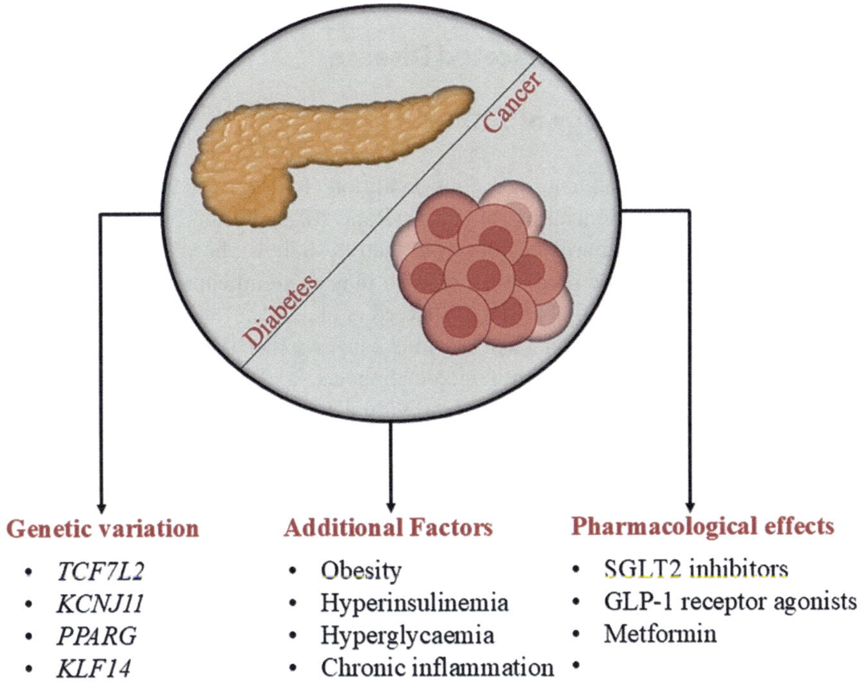

Fig. 1 Risk factors associated with cancer and diabetes. This figure illustrates the interplay between diabetes and cancer, emphasizing key contributing factors. Genetic variations such as TCF7L2, KCNJ11, PPARG, and KLF14 are associated with diabetes susceptibility. Additional risk factors, including obesity, hyperinsulinemia, hyperglycemia, and chronic inflammation, further exacerbate disease progression. Pharmacological interventions like SGLT2 inhibitors, GLP-1 receptor agonists, and metformin play a crucial role in managing diabetes while potentially influencing cancer risk. SGLT2 inhibitors sodium-glucose cotransporter-2, GLP-1 glucagon-like peptide 1

diseases. By acknowledging the interconnectedness between diabetes and cancer, patient outcomes can be improved through more efficient management strategies that address the complexities of these chronic diseases.

Objectives
This chapter aims to elucidate the connection between diabetes and cancer as follows:

- Exploring the epidemiological evidence linking diabetes to cancer.
- Examining the underlying biological mechanisms of this association.
- Discussing shared risk factors that contribute to increased cancer incidence among diabetic patients.
- Reviewing present treatment protocols for managing patients with both conditions.
- Emphasizing the need for integrated care approaches addressing both diseases simultaneously.

2 Diabetes: A Multifaceted Disease

2.1 Pathophysiology of T2D

T2D is a multifaceted and heterogeneous condition characterized by chronic hyperglycemia and inadequate insulin production (Raja, 2023). Formerly known as adult-onset diabetes, T2D primarily results from factors such as obesity and a sedentary lifestyle, although genetic predisposition also plays a significant role. It represents approximately 90% of all diabetes cases (Reed et al., 2021).

T2D is a group of disorders with various causes rather than one illness. These include polygenic influences, monogenic diabetes, and pathophysiological processes (Prasad & Groop, 2015). Each individual with T2D may present a unique combination of these factors with differing degrees of severity. Some individuals may primarily experience severe beta cell dysfunction, whereas others may have predominant insulin resistance.

2.2 Genetic Factors in T2D

Most cases of T2D are polygenic, meaning they involve multiple genetic and environmental interactions (Tremblay & Hamet, 2019). However, some rare forms of diabetes are monogenic, which means that mutations in a single gene can cause them. One example of a genetic condition is maturity-onset diabetes of the young (MODY), which comprises several subtypes linked to specific gene mutations, such as GCK, HNF1A, and HNF4A (Zečević et al., 2024). Although many MODY subtypes are mostly related to diabetes, MODY type 5 is also linked to renal cysts, and MODY type 8 is connected to exocrine pancreatic malfunction (Murphy et al., 2008).

2.3 Complications of T2D

Various complications, such as microvascular, macrovascular, and neuropathy, may arise from poorly controlled T2D. Small blood artery damage causes microvascular problems affecting the kidneys, nerves, and retina. Large blood arteries are involved in macrovascular issues, which may increase the risk of cardiovascular illnesses. Neuropathic complications affect nerves, leading to peripheral and autonomic neuropathy. T2D is associated with a higher probability of cognitive dysfunction, dementia, and specific infections (Chellaiyan et al., 2022). The cardiovascular risk associated with diabetes is likely due to insulin resistance, which often includes lipid abnormalities such as elevated small, dense LDL cholesterol particles and low HDL cholesterol levels (Hirano, 2018). Hypertension also contributes to these risks.

3 Cancer: A Complex Group of Diseases

Cancer includes a range of diseases marked by abnormal cellular proliferation, the potential to invade nearby tissues, and the ability to spread to distant organs (P. K. C. Sekar et al., 2024). It typically arises from genetic mutations and epigenetic alterations that interfere with standard cellular functions, including cell cycle regulation and immune surveillance. Although cancer can affect any part of the body, certain types are more prevalent and result in higher mortality rates (Coyle et al., 2017).

3.1 Hallmarks of Cancer: Uncontrolled Growth, Metastasis, and Immune Evasion

Hanahan and Weinberg defined the hallmarks of cancer as the biological capabilities acquired by cancer cells during tumor progression (Hanahan & Weinberg, 2011):

- *Uncontrolled growth*: Cancer cells evade growth suppressors and sustain proliferative signaling, leading to unchecked cell division. Unlike normal cells, which respond to signals regulating growth, cancer cells can activate oncogenes (e.g., RAS and MYC) and inactivate tumor suppressor genes (e.g., TP53 and RB1), allowing continuous proliferation. For example, in colorectal cancer, mutations in APC lead to dysregulated Wnt signaling and excessive cellular proliferation (Amin et al., 2015).
- *Metastasis*: Cancer cells acquire the capacity to infiltrate adjacent tissues and disseminate to distant organs through the bloodstream. A key process in this process is epithelial-mesenchymal transition (EMT), which enhances tumor cells' migratory and invasive characteristics. For example, breast cancer frequently metastasizes to the bones and lungs, mainly due to the increased expression of matrix metalloproteinases (MMPs) that break down extracellular matrix barriers (Banyard & Bielenberg, 2015).

- *Immune evasion*: Cancer cells employ multiple strategies to evade immune surveillance, including upregulating immune checkpoint proteins (e.g., PD-L1 and CTLA-4) that suppress T-cell function (Buchbinder & Desai, 2016). Lung cancer frequently exploits this mechanism, which leads to immune evasion and rapid disease progression. Immune checkpoint inhibitors such as pembrolizumab (anti-PD-1) have been developed to counteract this evasion and restore immune function against tumors.

3.2 Common Cancers: Breast, Prostate, Colorectal, and Lung

Certain cancers have high global incidence and mortality rates. Among the most significant are breast, prostate, colorectal, and lung cancers due to their prevalence. Lung cancer was the predominant cause of cancer mortality, accounting for 18.7% of total cancer deaths, followed by colorectal cancer (9.3%), liver cancer (7.8%), breast cancer (6.9%), and stomach cancer (6.8%) (Bray et al., 2024):

- *Breast cancer*: Breast cancer arises from ductal or lobular epithelium. The subtypes include HR+, HER2-positive, and triple-negative breast cancers. BRCA1/BRCA2 mutations increase susceptibility (Yersal & Barutca, 2014).
- *Prostate cancer*: A leading cancer in men, prostate cancer is primarily androgen-dependent, with AR playing a key role in disease progression (Yamada & Beltran, 2021). They can range from slow-growing tumors to aggressive and metastatic forms.
- *Colorectal cancer (CRC)*: CRC typically develops from adenomatous polyps and progresses through an adenoma-carcinoma sequence. Lynch syndrome, resulting from mutations in the MLH1 and MSH2 genes, increases the risk of CRC (Armaghany et al., 2012).
- *Lung cancer is* the most prevalent cause of cancer-related death. Non-small cell lung cancer (NSCLC) and small cell lung cancer (SCLC) are two primary subtypes. Smoking is the leading risk factor for lung cancer development. EGFR, ALK, and KRAS mutations induce cancer development (Tseng et al., 2017).

3.3 Cancer Risk Factors: Genetics, Lifestyle, and Environmental Factors

Cancer development is influenced by intricate interactions between genetic factors, environmental factors, and lifestyle choices (Parsa, 2012). Recognizing and managing these risk factors can significantly reduce the incidence of cancer. Hereditary mutations contribute to roughly 5–10% of all cancer cases (Hart et al., 2020). Mutations in BRCA1 and BRCA2 are associated with an elevated risk of breast and ovarian cancers (Jara et al., 2017), while TP53 mutations, associated with Li-Fraumeni syndrome (Guha & Malkin, 2017), predispose individuals to various types of cancer. Advances in genetic screening have enabled early detection and preventive measures such as prophylactic mastectomy for high-risk individuals.

Major modifiable risk factors include poor dietary habits, obesity, lack of physical activity, and alcohol and tobacco consumption. Additionally, exposure to environmental carcinogens significantly influences the risk of cancer.

4 Shared Pathophysiological Mechanisms

Diabetes and cancer share several underlying pathophysiological mechanisms that contribute to their co-occurrence and increased risk (Zhu & Qu, 2022). These shared mechanisms include chronic inflammation, dysregulation of insulin, oxidative stress, and immune dysfunction (Xu, 2014). Comprehending these interconnected pathways is necessary to create efficient prevention and treatment strategies that address both conditions. Table 2 represents the pathophysiological mechanisms between diabetes and cancer.

4.1 Chronic Inflammation: A Key Link

Chronic inflammation is a key characteristic of diabetes and cancer, establishing a critical association between them (Tsalamandris et al., 2019). Chronic low-grade inflammation is often associated with insulin resistance in diabetes. Inflammation can promote tumor initiation, growth, and metastasis. Several factors contribute to chronic inflammation under both conditions (Arcidiacono et al., 2012).

4.1.1 Role of Adipose Tissue and Macrophages

Visceral fat in adipose tissue is key to chronic inflammation (Kawai et al., 2021). In obesity, adipose tissue infiltrates immune cells, including macrophages, contributing to a proinflammatory state. Adipose tissue macrophages (ATMs) are essential in

Table 2 Shared pathophysiological mechanisms between diabetes and cancer

Mechanism	Role in diabetes	Role in cancer	Impact on disease progression
Chronic inflammation	Persistent low-grade inflammation due to insulin resistance	Promotes tumor initiation	Increased risk of cancer in diabetic individuals
Hyperinsulinemia	Elevated insulin levels due to insulin resistance	IGF-1 enhances cancer cell proliferation	Supports tumor growth
Oxidative stress	Hyperglycemia-induced production of ROS damages cells	Genomic instability led to tumorigenesis	Accelerates cancer development in diabetic patients
Immune dysfunction	Impaired immune surveillance due to chronic hyperglycemia	Cancer cells evade immune detection	Reduced ability to eliminate cancer cells in diabetic patients

producing inflammatory cytokines, including TNF-α and IL-6, which are implicated in insulin resistance and systemic inflammation and are essential for producing inflammatory cytokines. ATMs can be classified into two types: M1 and M2. M1 macrophages secrete proinflammatory mediators, whereas M2 macrophages release anti-inflammatory mediators that help maintain insulin sensitivity. Obesity induces M1 macrophages to secrete TNF-α, IL-6, IL-12, IL-1β, and other proinflammatory factors, resulting in inflammation and insulin resistance (Liang et al., 2022). For example, in colorectal cancer, obesity-induced inflammation upregulates NF-κB signaling, promoting tumor growth through increased cytokine production and epithelial proliferation (Kolb et al., 2016).

4.1.2 Cytokine Signaling and Insulin Resistance

The inflammatory cytokines ATMs and other immune cells release interfere with insulin signaling, leading to insulin resistance (de Luca & Olefsky, 2008). TNF-α, for example, can activate signaling pathways that inhibit the insulin receptor substrate (IRS), impairing the ability of insulin to stimulate glucose uptake in target tissues. IL-6 can also promote insulin resistance by activating the SOCS pathway, which inhibits insulin signaling. Furthermore, chronic inflammation can disrupt the balance between adipokines and hormones secreted by the adipose tissue (Clemente-Suárez et al., 2023). Chronic inflammation can result from prolonged activation of the innate immune system and is linked to several diseases, including T2D. Low-grade inflammation increases the risk of developing T2D, whereas subclinical inflammation contributes to insulin resistance. This condition is associated with the characteristics of metabolic syndrome, including elevated blood sugar levels (Badawi et al., 2010). For example, in hepatocellular carcinoma (HCC), chronic insulin resistance increases IGF-1 levels and promotes hepatocyte proliferation and survival, ultimately predisposing individuals to liver cancer (Shan et al., 2022).

4.2 Insulin and Insulin-Like Growth Factors: Impact on Cell Growth and Proliferation

Insulin and insulin-like growth factors (IGFs) are critical regulators of cell growth and metabolism (LeRoith et al., 2011). In diabetes, particularly T2D, insulin resistance often leads to hyperinsulinemia, in which the pancreas produces excess insulin to compensate for reduced insulin sensitivity. Elevated levels of insulin and IGFs can promote cancer development via several mechanisms. Insulin IGF-1 and IGF-II levels are linked with tumor growth (Gallagher & LeRoith, 2010). By activating the PI3K/Akt/mTOR pathway, which controls cell growth, survival, and metabolism, insulin signaling in cancer cells may promote tumor development and metastasis (Gallagher & LeRoith, 2010). IGFs are essential for cell development and proliferation, particularly IGF-1. IGF-1 signaling via IGF-1R activates downstream pathways analogous to insulin, facilitating tumor growth and survival. IGFs may also promote angiogenesis, a process that produces new blood vessels and is essential for developing and spreading tumors. The link between obesity, T2D, and cancer may be related, in part, to hyperinsulinemia secondary to insulin resistance (A. M. Y. Zhang et al., 2021).

4.3 Oxidative Stress: DNA Damage and Tumorigenesis

Oxidative stress is the disparity between producing reactive oxygen species (ROS) and the body's antioxidant defense. This mechanism is also shared between diabetes and cancer (Caturano et al., 2023). In diabetes, hyperglycemia contributes to elevated ROS production via multiple mechanisms, such as glucose auto-oxidation and the production of advanced glycation end products (AGEs). Excessive production of ROS can impair cellular components such as DNA and lipids, resulting in cellular dysfunction. Oxidative stress-induced DNA damage can promote cancer development by causing mutations, genomic instability, and altered gene expression (Dizdaroglu, 2015). DNA damage is a common characteristic of carcinogenesis and is elevated in patients with T2D. This increase was attributed to the higher production of reactive oxygen species and lower antioxidant capacity (Lee & Chan, 2015). For example, oxidative stress can lead to the formation of DNA adducts, a marker of oxidative DNA damage, which can cause mutations if not repaired (Pilger & Rüdiger, 2006). Oxidative stress can activate signaling pathways that encourage cell proliferation and contribute to tumor development. Oxidative stress is likely the primary factor mediating DNA damage in diabetes. This DNA damage can lead to crucial mutations in carcinogenesis (Arfin et al., 2021).

4.4 Immune Dysfunction: Impaired Cancer Surveillance

Immune dysfunction is increasingly acknowledged as a significant factor in diabetes and cancer (Berbudi et al., 2020). In diabetes, chronic inflammation and metabolic dysregulation can impair immune cell function, leading to reduced ability to fight infections and increased susceptibility to cancer. For example, hyperglycemia can impair the function of neutrophils, macrophages, and T-cells, reducing their ability to eliminate pathogens and tumor cells. Furthermore, diabetes-associated immune dysfunction can compromise cancer surveillance (Zhao et al., 2021). The decreased cytotoxic activity of natural killer cells and compromised T-cell responses facilitate the evasion of cancer cells from immune surveillance, thereby enhancing tumor growth and metastasis. Checkpoint inhibitors in cancer therapy induce insulin-dependent diabetes (Ghazvinian et al., 2023). Figure 2 depicts the shared pathophysiology between cancer and diabetes.

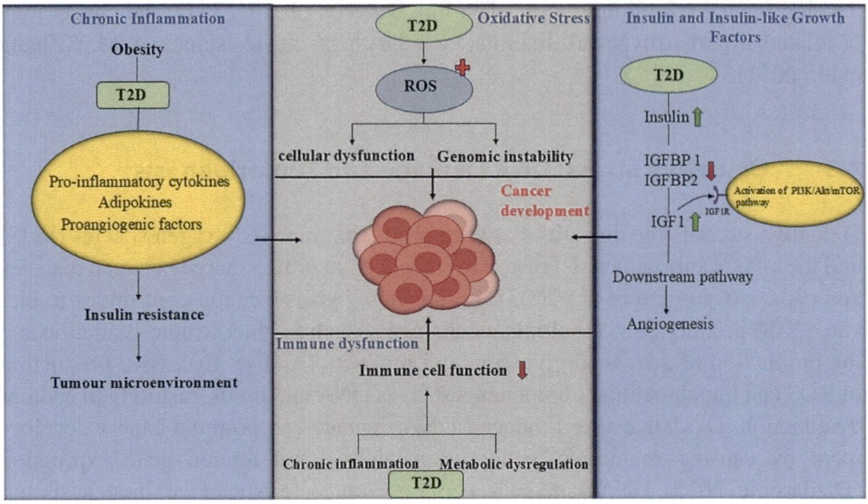

Fig. 2 Common pathophysiological mechanisms linking diabetes and cancer. This figure illustrates the complex interplay between T2D and cancer development through mechanisms involving chronic inflammation, oxidative stress, and insulin/insulin-like growth factors. Obesity-induced chronic inflammation releases proinflammatory cytokines, adipokines, and proangiogenic factors, contributing to insulin resistance and a tumor-promoting microenvironment. Oxidative stress, driven by ROS, induces cellular dysfunction and genomic instability, further facilitating cancer progression. Elevated insulin levels and dysregulated IGF signaling also activate the PI3K/Akt/mTOR pathway, promoting downstream angiogenesis and tumor growth. T2D type 2 diabetes, ROS reactive oxygen species, IGFBP2 insulin-like growth factor binding protein 2, IGF1R-insulin-like growth factor 1 receptor

5 Diabetes and Cancer Risk

T2D is associated with an increased risk of various cancers (Vulichi et al., 2022). This increased risk is not solely due to shared risk factors, such as obesity, but also involves complex biological mechanisms (Safaei et al., 2021).

5.1 Increased Cancer Risk in Diabetes: Evidence and Mechanisms

Epidemiological studies have demonstrated a significant link between diabetes and increased risk of several cancer types. A comprehensive meta-analysis showed that T2D is associated with an approximately 10% increased risk of developing cancer (K. Tsilidis et al., 2015b). The relative risk for certain types of cancers, such as liver, pancreatic, and endometrial, ranges from 2.0 to 2.5. For other cancers, including breast, colon, and bladder cancers, the relative risk is between 1.2 and 1.5 in individuals with diabetes (Giovannucci et al., 2010). Even a slight increase in cancer risk due to DM can have significant consequences at the population level, given the growing global prevalence of diabetes. The National Cancer Institute (NCI) and ADA recognize diabetes as an independent risk factor for cancer (Giovannucci et al., 2010).

Various factors contribute to the enhanced risk of cancer in individuals with diabetes, and insulin resistance in T2D often leads to hyperinsulinemia, as the pancreas attempts to compensate for reduced insulin sensitivity. Elevated insulin levels can act as a growth factor, stimulating cell proliferation and inhibiting apoptosis, potentially promoting tumor growth and metastasis. Insulin activates PI3K/Akt/mTOR (Orgel & Mittelman, 2013). Hyperinsulinemia can increase IGF-1 production, increasing the risk of colorectal, lung, premenopausal breast, and prostate cancer. IGF-1 stimulates cancer cell proliferation and its capacity to spread. Hyperglycemia, a hallmark of diabetes, can favor tumorigenesis through the "Warburg effect," in which cancer cells rely on glycolysis for energy production (Iacobini et al., 2023). Figure 3 illustrates the factors that increase cancer risk in individuals with diabetes.

This increased glucose uptake by cancer cells can meet their proliferation requirements. T2D is often associated with chronic inflammation, which can create a microenvironment that promotes tumor cell growth, enhances metastasis, increases angiogenesis, and impairs the function of natural killer cells and macrophages. Hyperglycemia can increase superoxide production and oxidative stress, leading to mutations that contribute to tumorigenesis (González et al., 2023).

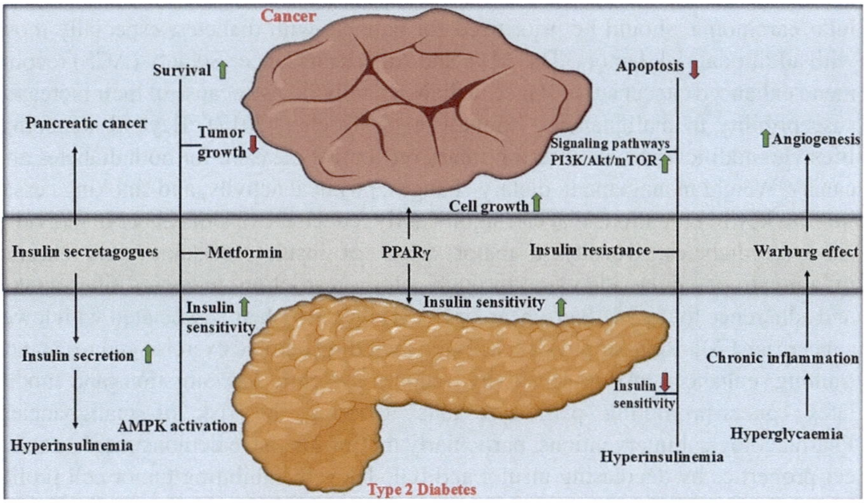

Fig. 3 Common factors contribute to the increased risk of cancer in individuals with diabetes. This figure highlights the shared molecular mechanisms that elevate cancer risk in individuals with T2D. Hyperinsulinemia, insulin resistance, and chronic inflammation create an environment that promotes tumor growth by enhancing insulin secretion, activating the PI3K/Akt/mTOR signaling pathway, and inducing angiogenesis. Additionally, the Warburg effect and high blood sugar levels (hyperglycemia) support tumor growth and survival while reducing programmed apoptosis

5.2 Specific Cancer Types: Breast, Pancreatic, Liver, and Colorectal

Research has indicated that individuals with T2D are at an increased risk of developing breast cancer (Eketunde, 2020). Specifically, African-American women with T2D may be at a higher risk of developing ER-negative breast cancer (Palmer et al., 2017). Additionally, the mortality rates among patients with diabetes were significantly higher in those with breast cancer. Individuals with newly diagnosed diabetes also have a greater risk of pancreatic cancer (Mellenthin et al., 2022). Hyperinsulinemia might possess an essential role in increasing the risk of pancreatic cancer among individuals with T2D. Furthermore, diabetes is linked with an elevated risk of liver cancer, and mortality rates among diabetes patients were significantly higher for liver cancer as well. Hyperglycemia is associated with an increased risk of colorectal cancer, and increased IGF-1 levels have been correlated with a greater risk of colorectal cancer (Zhao, 2024).

5.3 Preventive Strategies: Screening, Early Detection, and Lifestyle Modifications

Given the well-established association between diabetes and cancer risk, screening and early detection are critical for reducing cancer morbidity and mortality among individuals with diabetes. Routine cancer screenings, including mammography for breast cancer, colonoscopy for colorectal cancer, and liver ultrasound for hepatocellular carcinoma, should be prioritized for patients with diabetes, especially those with additional risk factors. The ADA and American Cancer Society (ACS) recommend enhanced cancer surveillance in diabetic individuals because of their increased susceptibility to malignancies (Mantovani & Targher, 2017). Beyond screening, lifestyle modifications serve as a primary preventive measure for both diabetes and cancer. Weight management, dietary changes, physical activity, and smoking cessation are key interventions that can significantly reduce the risk of cancer in individuals with diabetes. Obesity, a major driver of insulin resistance and chronic inflammation, can be addressed through caloric restriction, increased fiber intake, and adherence to the Mediterranean or DASH diet, which are associated with lower cancer risk [70]. Regular physical activity, including aerobic exercise and resistance training, enhances insulin sensitivity, reduces systemic inflammation, and modulates cancer-promoting pathways, thus lowering the risk of malignancies. Pharmacological interventions, particularly metformin, have demonstrated anticancer properties by decreasing insulin and IGF-1 levels, inhibiting tumor cell proliferation, and inducing apoptosis (Florkowski et al., 2024). Bariatric surgery in patients with severe obesity and T2D has been shown to reduce cancer incidence, likely due to its metabolic benefits, including improved insulin sensitivity and decreased inflammation. Finally, addressing modifiable risk factors, including smoking and alcohol consumption, is essential as both are independent risk factors for cancer and can worsen metabolic dysfunction in individuals with diabetes.

6 Lifestyle and Metabolic Interventions to Reduce Cancer Risk in Diabetes

Given the increased risk of cancer in individuals with diabetes, implementing lifestyle and metabolic interventions is crucial for reducing cancer risk. These interventions encompass dietary modifications, weight management, physical activity, and, when necessary, pharmacological strategies to improve glycemic control and overall metabolic health (Uusitupa et al., 2019).

6.1 Role of Diet: Nutritional Approaches and Glycemic Control

Diet significantly influences diabetes management and cancer risk (Ley et al., 2014). Nutritional approaches should focus on achieving optimal glycemic control, reducing inflammation, and promoting a healthy weight. A diet centered on plant-based foods, including vegetables, fruits, whole grains, and legumes, is advised. These foods are rich in fiber, vitamins, and antioxidants that can protect against cellular damage and reduce inflammation. Aim for at least 14 g of fiber per 1000 calories. Limit red meat intake to 12–18 ounces per week and avoid processed meats entirely (Aykan, 2015). Consume healthy fats from sources such as nuts and olive oil. Sugary drinks and refined carbohydrates can lead to elevated blood sugar levels and insulin resistance, thereby increasing the risk of cancer. A dietary pattern that includes high amounts of cereal fiber, coffee, fruits, and nuts and a high ratio of polyunsaturated fats to saturated fats and GI foods may help reduce the risk of breast cancer. Additionally, this pattern is characterized by a low intake of red and processed meats, sweetened beverages, and fruit juice. Maintaining stable blood sugar levels is crucial for reducing cancer risk. Choose foods with a low GI to prevent spikes in blood sugar.

6.2 Weight Management: Obesity and Cancer Prevention in Diabetic Individuals

Obesity is a well-known risk factor for diabetes and cancer. Excess body fat leads to chronic inflammation and hormonal imbalance, creating an environment that promotes tumor development. Adipose tissue secretes proinflammatory cytokines, including TNF-α, IL-6, and IL-1β, which can increase cancer cell growth and help cancer cells evade the immune system (Divella et al., 2016). Therefore, maintaining a healthy BMI and reducing visceral fat is essential to lower the risk of complications related to diabetes and cancer.

6.3 Physical Activity and Exercise: Improving Insulin Sensitivity and Immune Function

Interactions in physical activity are crucial for diabetes management and contribute significantly to cancer prevention. Regular exercise enhances insulin sensitivity and strengthens immune function (Vetrivel Venkatasamy et al., 2013). Attempt at least 150 min of moderate-intensity activity or 75 min of vigorous-intensity exercise each week.

6.4 Pharmacological Strategies

In addition to lifestyle changes, certain antidiabetic medications have shown potential anticancer properties through various mechanisms, such as reducing hyperinsulinemia, inhibiting cancer cell proliferation, and enhancing immune function. Metformin is a first-line medication for T2D that improves insulin sensitivity and lowers blood sugar levels. Research indicates that metformin is associated with a decreased risk of different types of cancers, including colorectal, breast, and prostate cancer. For example, one study found that cancer was diagnosed in 7.3% of metformin users compared to 11.6% of those who did not administer the drug (Sahra et al., 2010). SGLT2 inhibitors lower blood sugar levels by increasing glucose excretion in the urine. While preclinical studies have indicated that SGLT2 inhibitors may have potential anticancer effects (De Boer et al., 2022), additional research is needed to validate these findings. GLP-1 receptor agonists help to lower blood sugar levels. Preliminary evidence suggests that GLP-1 receptor agonists may possess anti-inflammatory and anticancer properties; however, additional studies are required to validate these claims. Although these pharmacological interventions promise to reduce cancer risk, longitudinal studies are needed to confirm their effectiveness in cancer prevention.

7 Diabetes Medications and Cancer Risk

The relationship between diabetes medications and cancer risk is complex and has been a subject of ongoing research. Although several studies have shown a correlation between certain diabetes drugs and an increased risk of cancer, others have indicated a protective effect, particularly with metformin (Johnson & Gale, 2010).

7.1 Insulin Therapy: Cancer Promotion Versus Neutral Effects

Insulin therapy is often necessary for managing hyperglycemia in individuals with diabetes; however, its impact on cancer risk has been a topic of debate. Some studies have suggested that high levels of insulin, whether from insulin resistance or exogenous insulin administration, could promote cancer cell growth and proliferation and can function as a growth factor by stimulating cell proliferation and inhibiting apoptosis through the activation of PI3K/Akt/mTOR signaling pathways (Johnson & Gale, 2010). However, other studies have found no significant association between insulin therapy and increased cancer risk (Hemkens et al., 2009). A key consideration is that the need for insulin therapy often reflects more advanced diabetes and poorer glycemic control, which are independently associated with an increased cancer risk. Therefore, it can be challenging to disentangle the direct effects of insulin from the impact of the underlying metabolic dysfunction. Recent research indicates that for those taking GLP-1RAs, no association was found to reduce the risk of breast cancer compared to those taking insulin (L. Wang et al., 2024).

7.2 Other Diabetes Medications and Their Influence on Cancer Risk

The impact of various diabetic medications on cancer risk remains uncertain and requires further research. A review conducted by researchers at Indiana University examined 46 clinical trials involving >34,000 patients. The findings indicated that individuals taking SGLT2 inhibitors did not have an increased risk of developing most types of cancer (Tang et al., 2017). A recent study found that GLP-1 receptor agonists such as Ozempic and Wegovy are not linked to an increased risk of pancreatic cancer (Ayoub et al., 2024). Furthermore, diabetes drugs such as GLP-1RAs may reduce the risk of ten cancers. Risks associated with stomach cancer in this comparison showed a hazard ratio of less than 1 for participants taking GLP-1, but this did not reach statistical significance. Some studies have suggested a possible increased risk of certain cancers, such as pancreatic cancer, with sulfonylurea use (Evans et al., 2005). However, the evidence remains inconsistent, and additional studies have not verified this association. It is crucial to emphasize that sulfonylureas can promote insulin secretion, potentially resulting in hyperinsulinemia that may contribute to cancer development.

8 Genetic and Epigenetic Links Between Diabetes and Cancer

The connection between cancer and diabetes has been apparent for decades, and recent research has begun to uncover the underlying genetic and epigenetic mechanisms contributing to this relationship.

8.1 Genetic Susceptibility to both Diseases

Genetic factors significantly influence susceptibility to T2D and various cancers (K. K. Tsilidis et al., 2015a). Numerous genes have been found to increase the probability of both ailments. GWAS have identified specific genetic variations that influence the onset of T2D and various malignancies. For instance, two particular genetic variants have been identified as key contributors to the risk of developing both T2D and some types of cancer. One variation correlates with an enhanced risk of breast cancer, while the other variant impacts the risks of breast, colorectal, and pancreatic cancers (Bonagiri & Shubrook, 2020). Furthermore, several studies suggested that HNF1B may be associated with an elevated risk of diabetes and a reduced risk of prostate cancer (Stevens et al., 2010). A study analyzing whole-genome sequencing data from childhood cancer survivors identified four novel risk loci for T2D, with three achieving genome-wide significance. These loci, which include variants of LINC02112, MYT1L, and ZNF492, showed evidence of modifying the risk of T2D related to alkylating agent therapy. In addition, some genetic variants may have a disproportionately large effect on individuals of specific ancestries. For example, the same study found that therapy-related genetic risks contribute to an increased burden of T2D among non-Hispanic black survivors (Im et al., 2024).

Polygenic risk scores, which combine the effects of multiple genetic variants, can be used to evaluate an individual's overall genetic risk of T2D. One study showed that polygenic risk scores developed from diverse ancestry datasets were more effective in assessing diabetes risk among individuals of both European and African ancestry (Redondo et al., 2022).

8.2 Epigenetic Modifications in Diabetes and Tumorigenesis

Both diabetes and cancer are influenced by epigenetic changes that change the expression of genes without altering the underlying DNA sequence. Elevated blood glucose levels, which are a symptom of diabetes, may contribute to the development of cancer. Hyperglycemia damages the body's DNA. High glucose levels can change the structure of DNA and inhibit its natural repair processes, which can cause instability in the genome and allow cancer cells to proliferate (Ling & Rönn, 2019). In people who are genetically predisposed to diabetes, alkylating agents, a family of chemotherapeutic medications, can increase their risk. According to the study, exposure to alkylating drugs, a type of chemotherapy frequently used in the treatment of cancer in children, may also increase the risk of developing type 2 diabetes (Meacham et al., 2009).

9 Cancer Treatment and Diabetes Management

The intersection of cancer treatment and diabetes management presents unique challenges owing to the potential impact of cancer therapies on glucose control and overall metabolic health. Chemotherapy, radiation therapy, and immunotherapy can affect diabetes management, necessitating careful strategies to mitigate adverse effects and optimize patient outcomes.

9.1 Impact of Cancer Treatments on Diabetes: Chemotherapy, Radiation, and Immunotherapy

Cancer treatments can significantly affect blood sugar levels and overall diabetes management. Chemotherapy, radiation, and immunotherapy have unique mechanisms that disrupt glucose homeostasis (Y. Zhang et al., 2022). Chemotherapy drugs can cause various side effects. Certain chemotherapy drugs, like asparaginase and busulfan, can directly raise blood sugar levels. Additionally, chemotherapy is often administered alongside steroids, which can further worsen hyperglycemia. Therefore, patients undergoing chemotherapy may need to adjust their diabetes medications accordingly. Radiation therapy, mainly when targeted at the abdomen or pancreas, can increase the risk of diabetes. Abdominal irradiation has been linked to decreased insulin secretion. Radiation pneumonitis, a common adverse reaction to radiation therapy for chest tumors, may occur more frequently in patients with diabetes. Furthermore, glucocorticoids, which are often used to treat radiation pneumonitis, can negatively affect blood glucose control, making diabetes management more complicated. Immunotherapy has transformed cancer treatment but can also cause immune-related adverse events, such as diabetes. Immune checkpoint inhibitors (ICIs) may lead to the development of new-onset diabetes, frequently manifesting as diabetic ketoacidosis. This condition arises from the immune-mediated destruction of pancreatic beta cells. In cases of immunotherapy-induced diabetes, traditional type 1 diabetes autoantibodies may be absent. Prompt insulin therapy and close collaboration between endocrinologists and oncologists are essential. Additionally, steroids, frequently used in conjunction with cancer treatments, can elevate blood sugar levels and potentially lead to steroid-induced diabetes, particularly in individuals with preexisting risk factors.

9.2 Managing Diabetes During Cancer Treatment: Challenges and Strategies

Patients with coexisting diabetes and cancer require comprehensive, multidisciplinary care to address both conditions simultaneously. Before initiating cancer treatment, assess the patient's glycemic control, diabetes medication regimen, and overall health status. Develop an individualized diabetes management plan that considers the specific cancer treatment, potential side effects, and the patient's ability to adhere to the plan. Encourage frequent self-monitoring of blood glucose levels to promptly detect and address hyperglycemia or hypoglycemia. Adjust diabetes medications as needed to maintain optimal glycemic control. Insulin dosages may need to be modified, and oral hypoglycemic agents may need to be temporarily discontinued or adjusted. Provide nutritional counseling to help patients manage their diet and maintain adequate nutrition despite treatment-related side effects. Encourage small, frequent meals and healthy snacks to prevent hypoglycemia. Ensure clear communication and coordination of care between the oncology and endocrinology teams to optimize diabetes management and cancer treatment outcomes (Silvestris et al., 2023).

9.3 Long-Term Consequences of Cancer Treatments on Diabetes

Cancer treatments can have long-term consequences on diabetes management, including persistent hyperglycemia, increased insulin resistance, and an elevated risk of diabetes-related complications (Skyler et al., 2017). Both diabetes and cancer treatments independently increase the risk of CVD (P. Sekar & Veerabathiran, 2024). Chemotherapy agents such as anthracyclines and tyrosine kinase inhibitors (TKIs) are known to cause cardiotoxicity, exacerbating the risk of heart disease in diabetic patients. Long-term surveillance for hypertension, dyslipidemia, and heart failure is essential in cancer survivors with diabetes. Radiation therapy targeting the pancreas can result in permanent beta cell damage, leading to insulin-dependent diabetes. Similarly, chemotherapy-induced beta cell toxicity can contribute to progressive insulin insufficiency over time. Regular assessment of pancreatic function and early intervention with insulin therapy may be necessary in affected individuals.

10 Conclusion

There is a complex relationship between diabetes and cancer. In summary, individuals with diabetes have a greater risk of developing various types of cancer and experience a higher mortality rate from cancer. Conversely, specific treatments for diabetes mellitus may also be correlated to an elevated risk of cancer. Several factors contribute to the link between diabetes and cancer. These include genetic predispositions, obesity, inflammation, high blood sugar, elevated insulin levels, cancer treatments, insulin use, and certain oral hypoglycemic medications. Given these associations, it is recommended that patients with diabetes undergo cancer screening and that special care is taken in managing diabetes for those diagnosed with cancer. Further research is necessary to deepen our understanding of the relationship between these two diseases.

Acknowledgments The authors thank the Chettinad Academy of Research Education for their constant support and encouragement.

References

American Diabetes Association. (2009). Diagnosis and classification of diabetes mellitus. *Diabetes Care, 32*(Suppl 1), S62–S67. https://doi.org/10.2337/dc09-S062

Amin, A. R. M. R., Karpowicz, P. A., Carey, T. E., Arbiser, J., Nahta, R., Chen, Z. G., Dong, J. T., Kucuk, O., Khan, G. N., Huang, G. S., Mi, S., Lee, H. Y., Reichrath, J., Honoki, K., Georgakilas, A. G., Amedei, A., Amin, A., Helferich, B., Boosani, C. S., et al. (2015). Evasion of anti-growth signaling: A key step in tumorigenesis and potential target for treatment and prophylaxis by natural compounds. *Seminars in Cancer Biology, 35*, S55–S77. https://doi.org/10.1016/J.SEMCANCER.2015.02.005

Arcidiacono, B., Iiritano, S., Nocera, A., Possidente, K., Nevolo, M. T., Ventura, V., Foti, D., Chiefari, E., & Brunetti, A. (2012). Insulin resistance and cancer risk: An overview of the pathogenetic mechanisms. *Experimental Diabetes Research, 2012*. https://doi.org/10.1155/2012/789174

Arfin, S., Kumar Jha, N., Kumar Jha, S., Kesari, K. K., Ruokolainen, J., Roychoudhury, S., Rathi, B., & Kumar, D. (2021). Oxidative stress in cancer cell metabolism. *Antioxidants, 10*(5). https://doi.org/10.3390/antiox10050642

Armaghany, T., Wilson, J., Chu, Q., & Mills, G. (2012). Genetic alterations in colorectal cancer. *Gastrointestinal Cancer Research*. Retrieved February 19, 2025, from https://www.ncbi.nlm.nih.gov/pmc/articles/PMC3348713/

Aykan, N. F. (2015). Red meat and colorectal cancer. *Oncology Reviews, 9*(1), 38–44. https://doi.org/10.4081/ONCOL.2015.288

Ayoub, M., Faris, C., Juranovic, T., Chela, H., & Cancers, E. D. (2024). The use of glucagon-like peptide-1 receptor agonists in patients with type 2 diabetes mellitus does not increase the risk of pancreatic cancer: A US-based Cohort. *Cancers, 16*(9). https://doi.org/10.3390/cancers16091625

Badawi, A., Klip, A., Haddad, P., Cole, D. E., Bailo, G., El-Sohemy, A., & Karmali, M. (2010). Type 2 diabetes mellitus and inflammation: Prospects for biomarkers of risk and nutritional intervention. *Diabetes, Metabolic Syndrome and Obesity: Targets and Therapy, 173*. https://doi.org/10.2147/dmsott.s9089

Banyard, J., & Bielenberg, D. R. (2015). The role of EMT and MET in cancer dissemination. *Connective Tissue Research, 56*(5), 403–413. https://doi.org/10.3109/03008207.2015.1060970

Berbudi, A., Rahmadika, N., Tjahjadi, A. I., & Ruslami, R. (2020). Type 2 diabetes and its impact on the immune system. *Current Diabetes Reviews, 16*(5), 442–449. https://doi.org/10.2174/1573399815666191024085838

Bonagiri, P. R., & Shubrook, J. H. (2020). Review of associations between type 2 diabetes and cancer. *Clinical Diabetes, 38*(3), 256–265. https://doi.org/10.2337/CD19-0077

Bray, F., Laversanne, M., Sung, H., Ferlay, J., Siegel, R. L., Soerjomataram, I., & Jemal, A. (2024). Global cancer statistics 2022: GLOBOCAN estimates of incidence and mortality worldwide for 36 cancers in 185 countries. *CA: A Cancer Journal for Clinicians, 74*(3), 229–263. https://doi.org/10.3322/CAAC.21834

Buchbinder, E. I., & Desai, A. (2016). CTLA-4 and PD-1 pathways similarities, differences, and implications of their inhibition. *American Journal of Clinical Oncology: Cancer Clinical Trials, 39*(1), 98–106. https://doi.org/10.1097/COC.0000000000000239

Caturano, A., D'Angelo, M., Mormone, A., Russo, V., Mollica, M. P., Salvatore, T., Galiero, R., Rinaldi, L., Vetrano, E., Marfella, R., Monda, M., Giordano, A., & Sasso, F. C. (2023). Oxidative stress in type 2 diabetes: Impacts from pathogenesis to lifestyle modifications. *Current Issues in Molecular Biology, 45*(8), 6651–6666. https://doi.org/10.3390/CIMB45080420

Chellaiyan, V. G., Jenniferbritto, J., & Alfred, J. (2022). Impact of digital health education among patients with type 2 diabetes mellitus. *National Journal of Community Medicine, 13*(03), 171–174. https://doi.org/10.55489/NJCM.1332022394

Clemente-Suárez, V. J., Redondo-Flórez, L., Beltrán-Velasco, A. I., Martín-Rodríguez, A., Martínez-Guardado, I., Navarro-Jiménez, E., Laborde-Cárdenas, C. C., & Tornero-Aguilera, J. F. (2023). The role of adipokines in health and disease. *Biomedicines, 11*(5). https://doi.org/10.3390/biomedicines11051290

Coyle, K. M., Boudreau, J. E., & Marcato, P. (2017). Genetic mutations and epigenetic modifications: Driving cancer and informing precision medicine. *BioMed Research International, 2017*. https://doi.org/10.1155/2017/9620870

De Boer, I. H., Khunti, K., Sadusky, T., Tuttle, K. R., Neumiller, J. J., Rhee, C. M., Rosas, S. E., Rossing, P., & Bakris, G. (2022). Diabetes management in chronic kidney disease: A consensus report by the American Diabetes Association (ADA) and kidney disease: Improving global outcomes. *Diabetes Care*. https://doi.org/10.2337/dci22-0027

de Luca, C., & Olefsky, J. M. (2008). Inflammation and insulin resistance. *FEBS Letters, 582*(1), 97–105. https://doi.org/10.1016/J.FEBSLET.2007.11.057

Dela Cruz, C. S., Tanoue, L. T., & Matthay, R. A. (2011). Lung cancer: Epidemiology, etiology, and prevention. *Clinics in Chest Medicine, 32*(4), 605–644. https://doi.org/10.1016/J.CCM.2011.09.001/ASSET/4719E4D9-F048-4077-B838-CED4F4AA5C01/MAIN.ASSETS/GR13.JPG

Divella, R., De Luca, R., Abbate, I., Naglieri, E., & Daniele, A. (2016). Obesity and cancer: The role of adipose tissue and adipo-cytokines-induced chronic inflammation. *Journal of Cancer, 7*(15), 2346–2359. https://doi.org/10.7150/JCA.16884

Dizdaroglu, M. (2015). Oxidatively induced DNA damage and its repair in cancer. *Mutation Research - Reviews in Mutation Research, 763*, 212–245. https://doi.org/10.1016/J.MRREV.2014.11.002

Eketunde, A. O. (2020). Diabetes as a risk factor for breast cancer. *Cureus*. https://doi.org/10.7759/CUREUS.8010

Evans, J. M. M., Donnelly, L. A., Emslie-Smith, A. M., Alessi, D. R., & Morris, A. D. (2005). Metformin and reduced risk of cancer in diabetic patients. *British Medical Journal, 330*(7503), 1304–1305. https://doi.org/10.1136/BMJ.38415.708634.F7

Florkowski, M., Abiona, E., Frank, K. M., & Brichacek, A. L. (2024). Obesity-associated inflammation countered by a Mediterranean diet: The role of gut-derived metabolites. *Frontiers in Nutrition, 11*. https://doi.org/10.3389/FNUT.2024.1392666/FULL

Gallagher, E. J., & LeRoith, D. (2010). The proliferating role of insulin and insulin-like growth factors in cancer. *Trends in Endocrinology and Metabolism, 21*(10), 610–618. https://doi.org/10.1016/J.TEM.2010.06.007

Gallagher, E. J., & LeRoith, D. (2015). Obesity and diabetes: The increased risk of cancer and cancer-related mortality. *Physiological Reviews, 95*(3), 727–748. https://doi.org/10.1152/PHYSREV.00030.2014/ASSET/IMAGES/LARGE/Z9J0031527270003.JPEG

Ghazvinian, Z., Abdolahi, S., Tokhanbigli, S., Tarzemani, S., Piccin, A., Reza Zali, M., Verdi, J., & Baghaei, K. (2023). Contribution of natural killer cells in innate immunity against colorectal cancer. *Frontiers in Oncology, 12*. https://doi.org/10.3389/FONC.2022.1077053/FULL

Giovannucci, E., Harlan, D. M., Archer, M. C., Bergenstal, R. M., Gapstur, S. M., Habel, L. A., Pollak, M., Regensteiner, J. G., & Yee, D. (2010). Diabetes and cancer: A consensus report. *Diabetes Care, 33*(7), 1674–1685. https://doi.org/10.2337/DC10-0666

González, P., Lozano, P., Ros, G., & Solano, F. (2023). Hyperglycemia and oxidative stress: An integral, updated and critical overview of their metabolic interconnections. *International Journal of Molecular Sciences, 24*(11), 9352. https://doi.org/10.3390/IJMS24119352

Guha, T., & Malkin, D. (2017). Inherited TP53 mutations and the Li–Fraumeni syndrome. *Cold Spring Harbor Perspectives in Medicine, 7*(4). https://doi.org/10.1101/cshperspect.a026187

Hanahan, D., & Weinberg, R. A. (2011). Hallmarks of cancer: The next generation. *Cell, 144*(5), 646–674. https://doi.org/10.1016/J.CELL.2011.02.013

Hart, S. N., Polley, E. C., Yussuf, A., Yadav, S., David, Goldgar, E., Hu, C., LaDuca, H., Smith, L. P., Fujimoto, J., Li, S., Couch, F. J., & Dolinsky, J. S. (2020). Mutation prevalence tables for hereditary cancer derived from multigene panel testing. *Human Mutation, 41*(8), e1–e6. https://doi.org/10.1002/humu.24053

Hemkens, L. G., Grouven, U., Bender, R., Günster, C., Gutschmidt, S., Selke, G. W., & Sawicki, P. T. (2009). Risk of malignancies in patients with diabetes treated with human insulin or insulin analogues: A cohort study. *Diabetologia, 52*(9), 1732–1744. https://doi.org/10.1007/s00125-009-1418-4

Hirano, T. (2018). Pathophysiology of diabetic dyslipidemia. *Journal of Atherosclerosis and Thrombosis, 25*(9), 771–782. https://doi.org/10.5551/JAT.RV17023

Iacobini, C., Vitale, M., Pugliese, G., & Menini, S. (2023). The "sweet" path to cancer: Focus on cellular glucose metabolism. *Frontiers in Oncology, 13*. https://doi.org/10.3389/FONC.2023.1202093/FULL

Im, C., Neupane, A., Baedke, J. L., Lenny, B., Delaney, A., Dixon, S. B., Chow, E. J., Mostoufi-Moab, S., Yang, T., Richard, M. A., Gramatges, M. M., Lupo, P. J., Sharafeldin, N., Bhatia, S.,

Armstrong, G. T., Hudson, M. M., Ness, K. K., Robison, L. L., Yasui, Y., et al. (2024). Trans-ancestral genetic risk factors for treatment-related type 2 diabetes mellitus in survivors of childhood cancer. *Journal of Clinical Oncology, 42*(19), 2306–2316. https://doi.org/10.1200/JCO.23.02281

Jara, L., Morales, S., De Mayo, T., Gonzalez-Hormazabal, P., Carrasco, V., & Godoy, R. (2017). Mutations in BRCA1, BRCA2 and other breast and ovarian cancer susceptibility genes in Central and South American populations. *Biological Research, 50*(1), 35. https://doi.org/10.1186/s40659-017-0139-2

Johnson, J. A., & Gale, E. A. M. (2010). Diabetes, insulin use, and cancer risk: Are observational studies part of the solution - Or part of the problem? *Diabetes, 59*(5), 1129–1131. https://doi.org/10.2337/DB10-0334

Kawai, T., Autieri, M. V., & Scalia, R. (2021). Adipose tissue inflammation and metabolic dysfunction in obesity. *American Journal of Physiology - Cell Physiology, 320*(3), C375–C391. https://doi.org/10.1152/AJPCELL.00379.2020

Kolb, R., Sutterwala, F. S., & Zhang, W. (2016). Obesity and cancer: Inflammation bridges the two. *Current Opinion in Pharmacology, 29*, 77–89. https://doi.org/10.1016/J.COPH.2016.07.005

Lee, S., & Chan, J. C. N. (2015). Evidence for DNA damage as a biological link between diabetes and cancer. *Chinese Medical Journal, 128*(11), 1543–1548. https://doi.org/10.4103/0366-6999.157693

LeRoith, D., Scheinman, E., & Bitton-Worms, K. (2011). The role for insulin and insulin-like growth factors in the increased risk of cancer in diabetes. *Rambam Maimonides Medical Journal, 2*(2). https://doi.org/10.5041/RMMJ.10043

Ley, S. H., Hamdy, O., Mohan, V., & Hu, F. B. (2014). Prevention and management of type 2 diabetes: Dietary components and nutritional strategies. *The Lancet, 383*(9933), 1999–2007. https://doi.org/10.1016/S0140-6736(14)60613-9

Liang, W., Qi, Y., Yi, H., Mao, C., Meng, Q., Wang, H., & Zheng, C. (2022). The roles of adipose tissue macrophages in human disease. *Frontiers in Immunology, 13*. https://doi.org/10.3389/FIMMU.2022.908749/FULL

Ling, C., & Rönn, T. (2019). Epigenetics in human obesity and type 2 diabetes. *Cell Metabolism, 29*(5), 1028–1044. https://doi.org/10.1016/J.CMET.2019.03.009

Mantovani, A., & Targher, G. (2017). Type 2 diabetes mellitus and risk of hepatocellular carcinoma: Spotlight on nonalcoholic fatty liver disease. *Annals of Translational Medicine, 5*(13). https://doi.org/10.21037/ATM.2017.04.41

Matheus, A. S. D. M., Tannus, L. R. M., Cobas, R. A., Palma, C. C. S., Negrato, C. A., & Gomes, M. D. B. (2013). Impact of diabetes on cardiovascular disease: An update. *International Journal of Hypertension, 2013*(1), 653789. https://doi.org/10.1155/2013/653789

Meacham, L. R., Sklar, C. A., Li, S., Liu, Q., Gimpel, N., Yasui, Y., Whitton, J. A., Stovall, M., Robison, L. L., & Oeffinger, K. C. (2009). Diabetes mellitus in long-term survivors of childhood cancer - Increased risk associated with radiation therapy: A report for the childhood cancer survivor study. *Archives of Internal Medicine, 169*(15), 1381–1388. https://doi.org/10.1001/ARCHINTERNMED.2009.209

Mellenthin, C., Balaban, V., Dugic, A., & Cullati, S. (2022). Risk factors for pancreatic cancer in patients with new-onset diabetes: A systematic review and meta-analysis. *Cancers, 14*(19). https://doi.org/10.3390/cancers14194684

Murphy, R., Ellard, S., & Hattersley, A. T. (2008). Clinical implications of a molecular genetic classification of monogenic β-cell diabetes. *Nature Clinical Practice Endocrinology & Metabolism, 4*(4), 200–213. https://doi.org/10.1038/ncpendmet0778

Ong, K. L., Stafford, L. K., McLaughlin, S. A., Boyko, E. J., Vollset, S. E., Smith, A. E., Dalton, B. E., Duprey, J., Cruz, J. A., Hagins, H., Lindstedt, P. A., Aali, A., Abate, Y. H., Abate, M. D., Abbasian, M., Abbasi-Kangevari, Z., Abbasi-Kangevari, M., ElHafeez, S. A., Abd-Rabu, R., et al. (2023). Global, regional, and national burden of diabetes from 1990 to 2021, with projections of prevalence to 2050: A systematic analysis for the Global Burden of Disease Study 2021. *The Lancet, 402*(10397), 203–234. https://doi.org/10.1016/S0140-6736(23)01301-6/ATTACHMENT/157D6ACF-4659-4C0A-AD9F-A912F471C2FF/MMC1.PDF

Orgel, E., & Mittelman, S. D. (2013). The links between insulin resistance, diabetes, and cancer. *Current Diabetes Reports, 13*(2), 213–222. https://doi.org/10.1007/S11892-012-0356-6

Palmer, J. R., Castro-Webb, N., Bertrand, K., Bethea, T. N., & Denis, G. V. (2017). Type II diabetes and incidence of estrogen receptor negative breast cancer in African American women. *Cancer Research, 77*(22), 6462–6469. https://doi.org/10.1158/0008-5472.CAN-17-1903

Parsa, N. (2012). Environmental factors inducing human cancers. *Iranian Journal of Public Health, 41*(11), 1–9.

Pilger, A., & Rüdiger, H. W. (2006). 8-Hydroxy-2′-deoxyguanosine as a marker of oxidative DNA damage related to occupational and environmental exposures. *International Archives of Occupational and Environmental Health, 80*(1), 1–15. https://doi.org/10.1007/S00420-006-0106-7

Prasad, R. B., & Groop, L. (2015). Genetics of type 2 diabetes—Pitfalls and possibilities. *Genes, 6*(1), 87–123. https://doi.org/10.3390/GENES6010087

Raja, D. (2023). From numbers to narratives: Understanding quality of life in type 2 diabetes. *Chettinad Health City Medical Journal, 12*(4), 1–2. https://doi.org/10.24321/2278.2044.202363

Redondo, M. J., Gignoux, C. R., Dabelea, D., Hagopian, W. A., Onengut-Gumuscu, S., Oram, R. A., & Rich, S. S. (2022). Type 1 diabetes in diverse ancestries and the use of genetic risk scores. *The Lancet Diabetes and Endocrinology, 10*(8), 597–608. https://doi.org/10.1016/S2213-8587(22)00159-0

Reed, J., Bain, S., & Kanamarlapudi, V. (2021). A review of current trends with type 2 diabetes epidemiology, aetiology, pathogenesis, treatments and future perspectives. *Diabetes, Metabolic Syndrome and Obesity, 14*, 3567–3602. https://doi.org/10.2147/DMSO.S319895

Safadi, H., Balogh, Á., Lám, J., Nagy, A., & Belicza, É. (2024). Associations between diabetes and cancer: A 10-year national population-based retrospective cohort study. *Diabetes Research and Clinical Practice, 211*, 111665. https://doi.org/10.1016/J.DIABRES.2024.111665

Safaei, M., Sundararajan, E. A., Driss, M., Boulila, W., & Shapi'i, A. (2021). A systematic literature review on obesity: Understanding the causes & consequences of obesity and reviewing various machine learning approaches used to predict obesity. *Computers in Biology and Medicine, 136*. https://doi.org/10.1016/J.COMPBIOMED.2021.104754

Sahra, I. B., Le Marchand-Brustel, Y., Tanti, J. F., & Bost, F. (2010). Metformin in cancer therapy: A new perspective for an old antidiabetic drug? *Molecular Cancer Therapeutics, 9*(5), 1092–1099. https://doi.org/10.1158/1535-7163.MCT-09-1186

Sekar, P., & Veerabathiran, R. (2024). The future of artificial intelligence and genetic insights in precision cardiovascular medicine: A comprehensive review. *Cardiology Discovery*. https://doi.org/10.1097/CD9.0000000000000136

Sekar, P. K. C., Thomas, S. M., & Veerabathiran, R. (2024). The future of cervical cancer prevention: Advances in research and technology. *Exploration of Medicine, 5*(3), 384–400. https://doi.org/10.37349/EMED.2024.00226

Shahid, R. K., Ahmed, S., Le, D., & Yadav, S. (2021). Diabetes and cancer: Risk, challenges, management and outcomes. *Cancers, 13*(22), 5735. https://doi.org/10.3390/CANCERS13225735

Shan, Y., Lu, C., Wang, J., Li, M., Ye, S., Wu, S., Huang, J., Bu, S., & Wang, F. (2022). IGF-1 contributes to liver cancer development in diabetes patients by promoting autophagy. *Annals of Hepatology, 27*(4). https://doi.org/10.1016/J.AOHEP.2022.100697

Silvestris, N., Franchina, T., Gallo, M., Argentiero, A., Avogaro, A., Cirino, G., Colao, A., Danesi, R., Di Cianni, G., D'Oronzo, S., Faggiano, A., Fogli, S., Giuffrida, D., Gori, S., Marrano, N., Mazzilli, R., Monami, M., Montagnani, M., Morviducci, L., et al. (2023). Diabetes management in cancer patients. An Italian Association of Medical Oncology, Italian Association of Medical Diabetologists, Italian Society of Diabetology, Italian Society of Endocrinology and Italian Society of Pharmacology multidisciplinary consensus position paper. *ESMO Open, 8*(6). https://doi.org/10.1016/J.ESMOOP.2023.102062

Skyler, J. S., Bakris, G. L., Bonifacio, E., Darsow, T., Eckel, R. H., Groop, L., Groop, P. H., Handelsman, Y., Insel, R. A., Mathieu, C., McElvaine, A. T., Palmer, J. P., Pugliese, A., Schatz, D. A., Sosenko, J. M., Wilding, J. P. H., & Ratner, R. E. (2017). Differentiation of diabetes by pathophysiology, natural history, and prognosis. *Diabetes, 66*(2), 241–255. https://doi.org/10.2337/DB16-0806

Stevens, V. L., Ahn, J., Sun, J., Jacobs, E. J., Moore, S. C., Patel, A. V., Berndt, S. I., Albanes, D., & Hayes, R. B. (2010). HNFIB and JAZFI genes, diabetes, and prostate cancer risk. *Prostate, 70*(6), 601–607. https://doi.org/10.1002/PROS.21094

Sung, H., Ferlay, J., Siegel, M. L., Soerjomataram, I., Jemal, A., & Bray, F. (2021). Global cancer statistics 2020: GLOBOCAN estimates of incidence and mortality worldwide for 36 cancers in 185 countries. *CA: A Cancer Journal for Clinicians, 71*(3), 209–249. https://doi.org/10.3322/caac.21660

Tang, H., Dai, Q., Shi, W., Zhai, S., Song, Y., & Han, J. (2017). SGLT2 inhibitors and risk of cancer in type 2 diabetes: A systematic review and meta-analysis of randomised controlled trials. *Diabetologia, 60*(10), 1862–1872. https://doi.org/10.1007/S00125-017-4370-8/FIGURES/4

Tremblay, J., & Hamet, P. (2019). Environmental and genetic contributions to diabetes. *Metabolism, 100*, 153952. https://doi.org/10.1016/J.METABOL.2019.153952

Tsalamandris, S., Antonopoulos, A. S., Oikonomou, E., Papamikroulis, G. A., Vogiatzi, G., Papaioannou, S., Deftereos, S., & Tousoulis, D. (2019). The role of inflammation in diabetes: Current concepts and future perspectives. *European Cardiology Review, 14*(1), 50–59. https://doi.org/10.15420/ECR.2018.33.1

Tseng, C. H., Chiang, C. J., Tseng, J. S., Yang, T. Y., Hsu, K. H., Chen, K. C., Wang, C. L., Chen, C. Y., Yen, S. H., Tsai, C. M., Huang, M. S., Ho, C. C., Yu, C. J., Tsai, Y. H., Chen, J. S., Chou, T. Y., Tsai, M. H., Chen, H. Y., Su, K. Y., et al. (2017). EGFR mutation, smoking, and gender in advanced lung adenocarcinoma. *Oncotarget, 8*(58), 98384–98393. https://doi.org/10.18632/ONCOTARGET.21842

Tsilidis, K. K., Allen, N. E., Appleby, P. N., Rohrmann, S., Nöthlings, U., Arriola, L., Gunter, M. J., Chajes, V., Rinaldi, S., Romieu, I., Murphy, N., Riboli, E., Tzoulaki, I., Kaaks, R., Lukanova, A., Boeing, H., Pischon, T., Dahm, C. C., Overvad, K., et al. (2015a). Diabetes mellitus and risk of prostate cancer in the European Prospective Investigation into Cancer and Nutrition. *International Journal of Cancer, 136*(2), 372–381. https://doi.org/10.1002/IJC.28989

Tsilidis, K., Kasimis, J., Lopez, D., Ntzani, E. E., & Ioannidis, J. P. A. (2015b). Type 2 diabetes and cancer: Umbrella review of meta-analyses of observational studies. *BMJ, 350*. https://doi.org/10.1136/bmj.g7607

Uusitupa, M., Khan, T. A., Viguiliouk, E., Kahleova, H., Rivellese, A. A., Hermansen, K., Pfeiffer, A., Thanopoulou, A., Salas-Salvadó, J., Schwab, U., Sievenpiper, J. L., & Li, K. (2019). Prevention of type 2 diabetes by lifestyle changes: A systematic review and meta-analysis. *Nutrients, 11*(11). https://doi.org/10.3390/nu11112611

Vetrivel Venkatasamy, V., Pericherla, S., Manthuruthil, S., Mishra, S., & Hanno, R. (2013). Effect of physical activity on insulin resistance, inflammation and oxidative stress in diabetes mellitus. *Journal of Clinical and Diagnostic Research, 7*(8), 1764–1766. https://doi.org/10.7860/JCDR/2013/6518.3306

Vulichi, S. R., Runthala, A., Begari, N., Rupak, K., Chunduri, V. R., Kapur, S., Chippada, A. R., & Sistla, D. S. M. (2022). Type-2 diabetes mellitus-associated cancer risk: In pursuit of understanding the possible link. *Diabetes & Metabolic Syndrome: Clinical Research & Reviews, 16*(9), 102591. https://doi.org/10.1016/J.DSX.2022.102591

Wang, L., Xu, R., Kaelber, D. C., & Berger, N. A. (2024). Glucagon-like peptide 1 receptor agonists and 13 obesity-associated cancers in patients with type 2 diabetes. *JAMA Network Open, 7*(7), e2421305–e2421305.

Wang, Y., Zeng, X., Tan, J., Xu, Y., & Yi, C. (2022). Diabetes mellitus and endometrial carcinoma: Risk factors and etiological links. *Medicine (United States), 101*(34), E30299. https://doi.org/10.1097/MD.0000000000030299

Xu, C.-X. (2014). Diabetes and cancer: Associations, mechanisms, and implications for medical practice. *World Journal of Diabetes, 5*(3), 372. https://doi.org/10.4239/WJD.V5.I3.372

Yamada, Y., & Beltran, H. (2021). Clinical and biological features of neuroendocrine prostate cancer. *Current Oncology Reports, 23*(2). https://doi.org/10.1007/S11912-020-01003-9

Yersal, O., & Barutca, S. (2014). Biological subtypes of breast cancer: Prognostic and therapeutic implications. *World Journal of Clinical Oncology, 5*(3), 412–424. https://doi.org/10.5306/WJCO.V5.I3.412

Zečević, K., Volčanšek, Š., Katsiki, N., Rizzo, M., Milardović, T. M., Stoian, A. P., Banach, M., & Muzurović, E. (2024). Maturity-onset diabetes of the young (MODY) - In search of ideal diagnostic criteria and precise treatment. *Progress in Cardiovascular Diseases, 85*, 14–25. https://doi.org/10.1016/J.PCAD.2024.03.004

Zhang, A. M. Y., Wellberg, E. A., Kopp, J. L., & Johnson, J. D. (2021). Hyperinsulinemia in obesity, inflammation, and cancer. *Diabetes and Metabolism Journal, 45*(3), 285–311. https://doi.org/10.4093/DMJ.2020.0250

Zhang, Y., Li, Q., Huang, Z., Li, B., Nice, E. C., Huang, C., Wei, L., & Zou, B. (2022). Targeting glucose metabolism enzymes in cancer treatment: Current and emerging strategies. *Cancers, 14*(19), 4568. https://doi.org/10.3390/CANCERS14194568

Zhao, H. (2024). Effect of hyperglycemia on the occurrence and prognosis of colorectal cancer. *American Journal of Translational Research, 16*(5), 2070–2081. https://doi.org/10.62347/NYHH3132

Zhao, H., Wu, L., Yan, G., Chen, Y., Zhou, M., Wu, Y., & Li, Y. (2021). Inflammation and tumor progression: Signaling pathways and targeted intervention. *Signal Transduction and Targeted Therapy, 6*(1). https://doi.org/10.1038/s41392-021-00658-5

Zhu, B., & Qu, S. (2022). The relationship between diabetes mellitus and cancers and its underlying mechanisms. *Frontiers in Endocrinology, 13*. https://doi.org/10.3389/FENDO.2022.800995/FULL

Inflammation and Oxidative Stress: Common Pathways in Diabetes and Cancer

Uthamalingam Murali, R. Muthuvel, Yupa Min, and Gowtham Kumar Subbaraj

Abstract

Diabetes mellitus and cancer, two of the most prevalent global health challenges, exhibit a complex interplay underpinned by shared pathological mechanisms. This abstract explores the intricate relationship between these seemingly distinct diseases, focusing on the pivotal roles of chronic inflammation and oxidative stress as common pathways that not only contribute to their individual pathogenesis but also foster their co-occurrence and mutual exacerbation. Metabolic dysregulation, a hallmark of diabetes, creates a milieu of hyperglycemia and insulin resistance, which in turn promotes the generation of reactive oxygen species (ROS) and the activation of pro-inflammatory signaling cascades. Similarly, the uncontrolled cellular proliferation characteristic of cancer is often accompanied by heightened metabolic activity, leading to increased oxidative stress and the release of inflammatory mediators that can fuel tumor growth, angiogenesis, and metastasis. The bidirectional link between diabetes and cancer is further evidenced by the observation that individuals with diabetes have an elevated risk of developing certain cancers, and conversely cancer and its treatments can impair glucose metabolism, increasing the likelihood of diabetes. This interconnectedness

U. Murali
Deparment of Surgery, Manipal University College Malaysia, Melaka, Malaysia

R. Muthuvel
Department of Biochemistry, Karuna Medical College and Hospital, Palakkad, Kerala, India

Y. Min
Department of Pathology, Faculty of Medicine, Quest International University, Ipoh, Malaysia

G. K. Subbaraj (✉)
Faculty of Allied Health Science, Chettinad Hospital and Research Institute, Chettinad Academy of Research and Education, Kelambakkam-603 103, Tamil Nadu, India

R. Noor (ed.), *Diabetes and Cancer: Association, Mechanism, and Therapeutic Implications*, https://doi.org/10.1007/978-981-95-5651-9_3

necessitates an integrated therapeutic approach that targets these shared underlying mechanisms. Strategies aimed at reducing chronic inflammation, improving metabolic regulation, and mitigating oxidative stress hold promise for both the prevention and management of these conditions. Emerging evidence suggests that lifestyle modifications, such as weight management and exercise, alongside certain antidiabetic medications like metformin, may exert beneficial effects on cancer risk, highlighting the potential for dual-targeting interventions.

Keywords

Diabetes mellitus · Cancer · Oxidative stress · Inflammation · Reactive oxygen species

1 Introduction

Many factors may induce inflammation, including infections brought on by microbial or viral agents, allergies, radiation, or harmful chemical substances; autoimmune or chronic disorders; obesity; strong alcohol or tobacco use; and a poor diet high in calories (Schetter et al., 2010; Aggarwal et al., 2009). Extended periods of inflammation are associated with an elevated risk of cancer. This inflammatory response can be classified as either acute or chronic. Immune system's activation mediates the first stage of inflammation (innate immunity), known as acute inflammation. This kind of inflammation is typically advantageous to the host and lasts just a brief period of time. When inflammation continues over a significant period, it transitions into chronic inflammation, which can elevate the risk of several long-term health issues, notably cancer (Lin & Karin, 2007). The recruitment of mast cells and leukocytes to the injury location during inflammation drives increased oxygen uptake, subsequently causing a surge in ROS production and accumulation at the damaged tissue, a process referred to as the "respiratory burst" (Hussain et al., 2003; Coussens & Werb, 2002).

An imbalance between the body's ability to produce free radicals and reactive oxygen species (ROS) and its antioxidant defenses leads to oxidative stress. This disruption can damage vital biomolecules and cells, potentially affecting the entire organism (Durackova, 2009). In addition to being waste products of regular cellular metabolism, reactive oxygen species (ROS) are essential for the activation of signaling pathways in plant and animal cells in reaction to changes in their environment (Jabs, 1999). In cells, reactive oxygen species (ROS) mostly come from the respiratory chain of mitochondria (Poyton et al., 2009). The metabolic breakdown of molecular oxygen in aerobic cells naturally produces these reactive oxygen species (ROS), which include organic peroxides, hydroxyl radicals, hydrogen peroxide, and superoxide anion (O2-) (Fridovich, 1978). The respiratory chain is where the electron transfer to molecular oxygen takes place, and the mitochondrial membranes contain the electron transport chains (Goossens et al., 1999; Goossens et al., 1995). Reactive nitrogen species (RNS) may be formed when oxygen is not present since nitric oxide (NO) is also produced by the mitochondrial respiratory chain (Poyton et al., 2009). These RNS may contribute to the production of extra reactive species including 4-hydroxynal (4-HNE) and malondialdehyde (MDA) by inducing excessive lipid peroxidation (Hussain et al., 2003). Additionally, important targets for oxidative assault are proteins and lipids, and altering these molecules can raise the risk of mutagenesis (Schraufstatter et al., 1988).

Diabetes and cancer are the most common and devastating illnesses of the contemporary period. In North America, diabetes affects around 10% of people, with type 2 diabetes accounting for nearly 95% of cases (Centers for Disease Control and Prevention, 2020; Liu et al., 2020). Endometrial, breast, colorectal, liver, and pancreatic cancers are among the many solid tumors that people with diabetes are more likely to acquire (Ling et al., 2020; Bjornsdottir et al., 2020). Cancer patients who also have diabetes present unique management challenges (Clore & Thurby-Hay, 2009). Diabetes mellitus appears to elevate the risk of specific cancer types. There is an elevated risk of both type 1 and type 2 diabetes (Cignarelli et al., 2018). Among those who have type 1 diabetes, cancer is the second most common killer (Livingstone et al., 2015). The concomitant use of steroids or a number of innovative cancer treatments may exacerbate preexisting diabetes or reveal underlying diabetes (Hughes et al., 2015; Morviducci et al., 2018). Studies have shown that individuals with diabetes exhibit an increased susceptibility to diverse illnesses and infection-related complications, leading to higher morbidity and mortality rates. Furthermore, cancer patients who also have diabetes demonstrate a greater risk of cancer-related mortality (Bjornsdottir et al., 2020; Coughlin et al., 2004; Saydah et al., 2003; Liu et al., 2012).

1.1 Unraveling the Molecular Culprits: Inflammation and Oxidative Stress

Oxidative stress and inflammatory mechanisms are major players in the diabetes-cancer relationship. An inflammatory microenvironment is created by chronic inflammation, which is characterized by elevated reactive oxygen species (ROS), abnormal adipokine production, pro-inflammatory pathway activation, high oxidative stress, and tumor growth, metastasis, angiogenesis, and macrophage and natural killer cell activity (Lin & Karin, 2007).

1.2 A Common Ground: Exploring Shared Pathophysiology

Diabetes, specifically type 2 diabetes, which is marked by insulin resistance and pancreatic β-cell dysfunction, has been linked metabolically to a number of malignancies, according to epidemiological studies. Diseases of the endometrium, ovaries, colon, pancreas, and bladder are more common in people with diabetes (Stevens et al., 2007; Shu et al., 2010). Signal transduction pathways that regulate nutrition utilization may be unbalanced, which could lead to the cancer risk linked to diabetes (Pollak, 2008).

The factors that underlie the correlation between diabetes and cancer are complex and often co-occur. Both insulin and glycemia at supraphysiological levels that are present in bodily tissues operate as powerful growth factors and sources of energy, respectively, that are necessary for the development of cancer and neoplastic transformation. Furthermore, hyperglycemia causes DNA damage and oxidative stress, which can start the initial stages of carcinogenesis (Calle & Kaaks, 2004; Ricart & Fernández-Real, 2001). Last but not least, regulatory bodies have been keeping an eye on a number of antihyperglycemic medications that were released in the past 10 years for potential increases in tumor incidence.

1.3 Inflammation: The Fuel for Disease

Inflammation plays a significant role in the relationship between cancer and diabetes mellitus (Balkwill & Mantovani, 2001). Type 2 diabetes is associated with inflammation-related irregularities in insulin secretion (American, 2021). Diabetes-related chronic inflammation can foster a milieu that is conducive to the growth of cancer. Obesity, which is frequently linked to a persistent subclinical inflammatory state, affects over 80% of T2D patients (Hotamisligil et al., 1993). Inflammation due to obesity and malfunctioning adipose tissue plays a major role in the association between diabetes, particularly type 2 diabetes, and the development of cancer (Balkwill & Mantovani, 2001).

1.4 Chronic Inflammation: A Silent Threat

An inflammatory microenvironment can be created by chronic inflammation, which is marked by increased reactive oxygen species (ROS), dysfunctional adipokine production, elevated oxidative stress, and enhanced tumor cell proliferation, metastasis, angiogenesis, and suppression of macrophage and natural killer cell function (Lin & Karin, 2007). The neoplastic process may be supported by a tumor-supporting microenvironment created by chronic inflammation (Lin & Karin, 2007), which is marked by elevated oxidative stress and ROS, aberrant adipokine synthesis, and pro-inflammatory pathway activation. Increased metastasis (IL-6, TGF-β, TNF-α), angiogenesis (IL-17, TGF-β, TNF-α), tumor cell development (IL-6, TNF-α), and impaired macrophage and natural killer cell activity have all been linked to particular cytokines produced from adipose tissue being present at higher levels (Lin & Karin, 2007).

1.5 The Immune System Gone Rogue: Inflammatory Mediators

Both diabetes and cancer are significantly influenced by inflammatory mediators, including cytokines and adipokines. By promoting inflammation, angiogenesis, and immune evasion mechanisms, these mediators aid in the development of cancer and contribute to insulin resistance in diabetes. The immunosuppressive ligand-receptor interaction-interfering checkpoint inhibitors (CPIs) have improved survival rates for an increasing number of cancer types and have therefore transformed cancer treatment (Azoury et al., 2015; Ribas & Wolchok, 2018). Immunological tolerance is maintained by checkpoint molecules such as cytotoxic T lymphocyte antigen 4 (CTLA-4) and programmed death 1 (PD-1) by inhibiting T cell activation (Pardoll, 2012). Aside from improving tumor cell destruction, monoclonal antibodies (mAbs) that target CTLA-4, PD-1, and its ligand, programmed death ligand 1 (PD-L1), have the potential to interfere with self-tolerance. This could lead to immune-related adverse events (irAEs) impacting different organ systems, such as autoimmune diabetes and pancreatic β-cells (Postow et al., 2018; Byun et al., 2017; De Velasco et al., 2017; Barroso-Sousa et al., 2018; Stamatouli et al., 2018; Chan & Bass, 2020; Quandt et al., 2020).

1.6 Inflammation's Role in Diabetes Development and Progression

Insulin secretory abnormalities linked to inflammation are linked to type 2 diabetes (American, 2021). The development of diabetes can be accelerated by inflammatory pathways that affect pancreatic beta-cell activity. Inflammation is considered a central element in the etiology of type 2 diabetes. Inflammatory mediators were shown to be a predictor of adult-onset type 2 diabetes in the early studies. Following this, further research found that higher plasma levels of C-reactive protein, interleukin-6, and sialic acid were linked to the development of type 2 diabetes mellitus in the future (Jesmin et al., 2010; Duncan, 2017). According to a different study, elevated inflammatory biomarkers were predictive of insulin resistance and type 2 diabetes development. An additional research, which looked at the correlation between diabetes patients' fasting insulin and C-reactive protein levels in plasma, brought attention to the link between the inflammatory pathways and insulin resistance (Schmidt et al., 1999; Pradhan et al., 2001).

The underlying cause of diabetic neuropathy is believed to be hyperglycemia-related metabolic, enzymatic, and microvascular changes that stimulate the formation of local and infiltrating pro-inflammatory cytokines and thus influence neurons in the CNS, PENS, and the autonomic nervous system (Navarro & Mora, 2005). Additionally, studies on animals have demonstrated that the retina of diabetic animals exhibits significantly increased levels of tumor necrosis factor-alpha and interleukin-1 mRNA expression in diabetic retinopathy and blocking this factor improves the disease's prevention (Pickup, 2004).

Dalla-Vestra et al. (Joussen et al., 2002) found that interleukin-6, fibrinogen, serum amyloid A, and C-reactive protein levels were all greater in patients with type 2 diabetes and nephropathy. Experimental evidence suggests that db/db mice, which mimic diabetes type 2 and diabetic nephropathy, have elevated levels of intracellular adhesion molecule-1, which is associated with inflammation by encouraging leukocyte and macrophage adherence and infiltration within the glomeruli and tubules (Dalla Vestra et al., 2005).

In type 2 diabetes mellitus, the inflammatory protein serum amyloid A may bind to the tanis gene, which has been identified as having expression that is dysregulated during fasting and significantly changed by glucose levels. The importance of the inflammation regarding the development of the illness is further supported by this discovery (Wander et al., 1994).

1.7 Inflammation's Contribution to Cancer Initiation and Growth

A favorable environment for the growth and spread of cancer cells is produced by inflammation. Angiogenesis, tumor development, and immune evasion are all facilitated by pro-inflammatory mediators and cytokines (Lin & Karin, 2007). Hyperglycemia and the inflammation it causes can harm tissue and encourage the development of cancer.

Oxidative stress and cancer are intimately related to inflammation. Persistent infections, autoimmune disorders, or environmental factors can cause chronic inflammation, which can lead to a pro-tumorigenic environment (Grivennikov et al., 2010). Neutrophils and macrophages, which are inflammatory cells, release ROS and RNS as a function of the immune response (Mittal et al., 2014). By causing harm to DNA and surrounding tissues, these reactive species can encourage mutations and genomic instability. Furthermore, signaling pathways supporting tumor growth and survival can be activated by inflammatory cytokines and chemokines generated by immune cells (Zhao et al., 2021). An inflammatory cytokine called tumor necrosis factor-alpha (TNF-α) may activate the nuclear factor κB (NF-κB) pathway and others that enable cell survival, especially in cancer cells (Wu & Zhou, 2010).

1.8 Oxidative Stress: The Rusting of Cells

A significant factor in the interaction between diabetes and cancer is oxidative stress. Insulin may promote the generation of ROS (Aggeli et al., 2011), whereas hyperglycemia may increase the creation of superoxide (Yu et al., 2006). Both stimulate signaling pathways that support carcinogenesis and cause damage to DNA (Valko et al., 2006). Individuals with diabetes often exhibit increased markers of oxidative stress (Navarro & Mora, 2005). This heightened oxidative environment can lead to cellular damage across various components, particularly DNA (Pickup, 2004). Since DNA mutations are a key factor in cancer development, the observation of elevated oxidative DNA damage indicators, such as 8-hydroxy-guanosine (8-OH-G), in diverse tumors suggests a strong association between this type of damage and the initiation of malignancies (Joussen et al., 2002). Hyperglycemia triggers the production of superoxide by the mitochondrial electron transport chain (Dalla Vestra et al., 2005). The ability of insulin to enhance reactive oxygen species (ROS) formation in skeletal myoblasts (Yu et al., 2006) and adipocytes (Wander et al., 1994) of obese individuals implies that hyperinsulinemia may worsen the oxidative stress seen alongside hyperglycemia (Hughes et al., 2015).

1.9 Free Radicals and Reactive Oxygen Species: The Double-Edged Sword

A key component of the etiology of both cancer and diabetes is oxidative stress, which generates free radicals and reactive oxygen species. ROS can harm DNA and other cellular constituents, causing mutations and accelerating the development of cancer.

The overproduction of ROS brought on by high glucose levels is the first step in hyperglycemia-induced oxidative damage. ROS are by-products of the autoxidation of glucose (González et al., 2023). Advanced glycation end products (AGEs) are a by-product of biological components such as proteins, lipids, nucleic acids, and reducing sugars, which are produced in a nonenzymatic process made possible by elevated glucose levels. Metal-catalyzed oxidation processes are one of the ways that AGEs produce ROS. Many tissues and organs may be severely impacted by this chain reaction of oxidative stress, which can result in cellular malfunction and damage (Khalid et al., 2022; Uceda et al., 2024).

The body's intricate antioxidant systems aim to neutralize reactive species; nevertheless, cancer may progress due to oxidative stress, which arises from an imbalance between the production of free radicals and antioxidant defenses (Lobo et al., 2010). Free radicals are implicated in cancer primarily through direct DNA damage (Sainz et al., 2012). The interaction on ROS and RNS with DNA leads to the base alterations, single- and double-strand breaks, and cross-linking. 8-Hydroxydeoxyguanosine (8-OHdG), a typical oxidative DNA lesion, results from ROS reacting with guanine bases (Santibáñez-Andrade et al., 2023). G to T transversions can result from 8-OHdG mispairing with adenine during DNA replication. Such mutations have the ability to turn healthy cells into cancerous ones if they arise in important genes such as tumor suppressor genes or oncogenes (Płachetka et al., 2013). For instance, many malignancies include mutations in the p53 tumor suppressor gene, which are usually brought on by oxidative stress (Rivlin et al., 2011).

1.10 Antioxidant Defense Mechanisms: Protecting Against Oxidative Damage

Glutathione, catalase, and superoxide dismutase are examples of antioxidant defense mechanisms that shield cells from oxidative damage. However, these systems might be overloaded when chronic oxidative stress is present, which would lead to cellular malfunction and the advancement of illness.

Dietary foods and drinks contain a variety of chemicals that alter cellular defenses and lower OS. Polyphenols, flavonoids, bioflavonoids, and many aromatic biophenols are among them (Fatima et al., 2018). Polyphenol-based dietary antioxidants can mitigate type 2 diabetes through two primary mechanisms: firstly, an insulin-dependent approach that safeguards and promotes pancreatic islet β-cell function by reducing oxidative stress and apoptosis, thereby enhancing insulin signaling and secretion, and, secondly, an insulin-independent strategy that involves reducing intestinal glucose uptake, inhibiting digestive enzyme activity, and regulating hepatic glucose release. Additionally, these antioxidants influence intracellular signaling pathways and gene expression (Shahwan et al., 2022).

Tumor cells can activate pathways that drive angiogenesis, proliferation, and metastasis and flourish in hypoxic environments when free radical levels are elevated (Amelio et al., 2014; Amelio & Melino, 2015; Amelio et al., 2015). Because high ROS levels increase the danger of oxidative stress-related damage, cancer cells frequently overexpress detoxifying proteins that increase their antioxidant capability. Cellular ROS scavengers are increased when the Nrf2 pathway is hyperactivated. Detoxifying force, which lowers stress burden, also influences several growth and proliferation-promoting pathways (Cho et al., 2015; Yadav et al., 2015; Singer et al., 2015). When cancer cells' antioxidant activity is blocked, their capacity to counteract oxidative damage is diminished, and cell death may ensue (Mei et al., 2015).

1.11 Oxidative Stress in Diabetes: A Vicious Cycle

Oxidative stress plays a substantial role in diabetes pathogenesis, as it impairs insulin secretion and intensifies insulin resistance. Furthermore, hyperglycemia can initiate a self-perpetuating cycle of oxidative damage by promoting reactive oxygen species (ROS) production, thus worsening the disease.

Oxidative stress plays a major role in the development of type 2 diabetes mellitus by triggering pro-inflammatory cytokines, hindering glucose utilization, insulin resistance, decreased insulin production, and dysregulated hepatic glucose metabolism (Rehman & Akash, 2017). Factors such as elevated glucose levels, hyperlipidemia, and inflammatory responses are recognized as sources of oxidative stress in pancreatic beta-cells (Dinarello et al., 2010). The subsequent rise in pro-inflammatory cytokine production, particularly tumor necrosis factor (TNF), is a direct result of this oxidative stress. Adipocytes also produce more reactive oxygen species, and oxidative stress caused by inflammation is thought to play a significant role in the development of type 2 diabetes (Donath et al., 2013).

It was recently demonstrated that oxidative stress is the primary cause of apoptosis in pancreatic beta-cells exposed to hyperglycemia and high amounts of free fatty acids (Piro et al., 2002). Additionally, oxidative stress biomarker measurements have been linked to pancreatic beta-cell lesions in type 2 diabetic volunteers, and patients with elevated oxidative stress have been shown to exhibit a marked decrease in antioxidant enzyme activity. The pathogenesis of type 2 diabetes is associated with autophagy initiated by oxidative stress. Specifically, free fatty acids, via lipid peroxidation, trigger autophagy in pancreatic beta-cells, causing insulin resistance in the periphery and oxidative stress, two hallmarks of the condition (Marciniak et al., 2004).

1.12 Oxidative Stress and Cancer: DNA Damage and Beyond

Gene expression and signal transduction pathways that are important in carcinogenesis are strongly impacted by oxidative stress (Valko et al., 2006). By triggering pro-inflammatory pathways including NF-κB, ROS have been shown to disrupt cell division and death (Valko et al., 2007). Reactive oxygen species (ROS) can induce a variety of DNA modifications, including base degradation; single- or double-stranded breaks; alterations in purine, pyrimidine, or sugar moieties; mutations; deletions; translocations; and protein cross-linking. Carcinogenesis, aging, and neurodegenerative, cardiovascular, and autoimmune illnesses are all significantly impacted by the majority of these DNA alterations. Redox metals, tobacco smoke, and nonredox metals including iron, cadmium, chrome, and arsenic all contribute to aging and carcinogenesis by forming free radicals or attaching themselves to thiol groups. The most well-known form of oxidative stress-induced DNA damage is the formation of 8-OH-G, which may be a biomarker for carcinogenesis (Valko et al., 2007).

1.13 The Interplay: Inflammation and Oxidative Stress in Diabetes and Cancer

Increased oxidative stress and persistent systemic inflammation go hand in hand with insulin resistance. The interplay between oxidative stress and inflammation, often termed "oxi-flammation," exerts influence over diverse cellular responses across various organ systems. Cardiovascular disorders, nephropathy, neuropathy, retinopathy, urological disorders, and cancer are among the consequences linked to diabetes that are influenced by the positive feedback cycle that involves oxidative stress, chronic systemic inflammation, and the development of insulin resistance (Harcourt et al., 2013; Malek et al., 2013; Vikram et al., 2010).

Inflammation and oxidative stress work hand in hand to cause cancer and diabetes. Because ROS and inflammatory cytokines affect insulin sensitivity and pancreatic function, they produce a microenvironment that promotes tumor growth and the advancement of diabetes.

1.14 A Dangerous Liaison: How Inflammation and Oxidative Stress Interact

The severity of diabetes and cancer is exacerbated by the combined effect of inflammation and oxidative stress. Risk on both diseases is increased by a vicious cycle in which ROS can activate inflammatory pathways and inflammatory mediators can encourage the generation of ROS.

Inflammation is a normal physiological response to many pathogenic occurrences, such as injury to tissues, invasion of microbes, and irritants. When damaged, cells from the immune system's innate and adaptive systems go to the site of the injury, activate, and secrete cytokines and other inflammatory mediators. It is believed that oxidative stress, which is caused by high glucose levels (Gumieniczek et al., 2005), facilitates the release of inflammatory mediators. Oxidative stress and chronic inflammation are known to have a significant role in the development of diabetes mellitus. Moreover, a close relationship exists between oxidative stress and inflammation in both normal and disease states (Ambade & Mandrekar, 2012).

Mechanisms for mutual amplification (also known as positive feedback or a "vicious cycle") are part of the intricate relationships between the oxidative stress and inflammatory pathways. The immune system's main response to viruses or other stimuli is inflammation, which helps cells return to normal or replace damaged tissue (Emmendoerffer et al., 2000). In response to stimuli from activated innate immune cells, the body releases cytokines and chemokines that promote inflammation and trigger the generation of reactive oxygen and nitrogen species (Emmendoerffer et al., 2000). In addition, by stimulating macrophage activation and the subsequent formation of reactive oxygen species, pro-inflammatory cytokines might indirectly induce oxidative stress (Miliara et al., 2015). Importantly, chronic inflammation is a long-term clinical disease that is characterized by fibrosis and tissue degradation. It ultimately leads to cell damage because inflammatory cells produce too many reactive oxygen species (ROS).

The detrimental cellular effects of chronic inflammation are primarily attributed to the sustained overproduction of free radicals and the depletion of antioxidant defenses (Fialkow et al., 2007). Reactive oxygen species (ROS) also contribute to inflammation by activating specific stress-activated kinases. Not only that, reactive oxygen species (ROS) have the ability to activate transcription factors like nuclear factor-kappa B (NF-kB) and activator protein-1 (AP-1), which in turn enhance the production of cytokines that cause inflammation. Thus, it would seem logical to propose that focusing on the oxidative stress-inflammatory cytokine signaling pathways would be a desirable approach to diabetes treatment. Immune system activation and oxidative stress are usually transient under normal physiological settings because of built-in regulation mechanisms such increased synthesis of antioxidant chemicals or anti-inflammatory cytokines. Both inflammation and oxidative stress are still active in some chronic disease states, including diabetes, and, depending on a number of variables, may have a beneficial or unfavorable effect on the management of the condition (Hold & El-Omar, 2008).

1.15 Signaling Pathways: The Messengers of Disease

Inflammation, oxidative stress, and cancer are all closely related to signaling pathways like NF-κB. Transcriptional regulation of genes involved in cell proliferation, survival, and metastasis is one manner in which these pathways impact diabetes and cancer progression.

One important intracellular mechanism, PI3K/AKT/mTOR, stimulates cell division, migration, and development while preventing tumor cells from undergoing apoptosis. PIP2 is changed into PIP3 by PI3K phosphorylation following activation by RTK binding. PTEN has a negative regulatory effect on this pathway. Following the recruitment of AKT and PDK1 to the plasma membrane, PDK1 phosphorylates AKT. After TSC2 is inactivated by this AKT phosphorylation, TSC1/TSC2 is degraded, and mTOR is activated, which results in mRNA translation, protein synthesis, and cell division.

Tumorigenesis is encouraged when these substances are activated. PI3K, AKT, and mTOR are inhibitory therapeutic targets. Several proteins and molecules are crucial to cellular signaling pathways, which are implicated in diabetes and cancer. Protein kinase B (Akt), mTORC1 and mTORC2, and phosphatase and tensin homolog (PTEN), which is located on chromosome 10, are among them. In addition, the following proteins are involved: receptor tyrosine kinase (RTK), phosphoinositide-dependent kinase 1 (PDK1), phosphoinositide-3-kinase (PI3K), triphosphatidylinositol 3,4,5-triphosphate (PIP3) and 4,5-bisphosphate (PIP2), and tuberous sclerosis proteins 1 and 2 (TSC1 and TSC2) (Asiri et al., 2024).

1.16 The Role of Genetics and Environmental Factors

The association between cancer and diabetes mellitus is likely influenced by a range of variables, such as genetic factors, obesity, inflammatory processes, oxidative stress, elevated glucose levels, high insulin levels, insulin, cancer treatments, and some oral hypoglycemic drugs.

1.17 Genetic Background

Genetic factors have been implicated in the development of both certain cancers and diabetes. For example, individuals with a familial history of pancreatic cancer often exhibit an increased susceptibility to the disease (Klein, 2012). Research has demonstrated a positive association between pancreatic cancer risk and specific glucose-elevating alleles, including those of FTO (rs8050136), MTNR1B (rs1387153), MADD (rs11039149) per allele, and glucokinase regulator (rs780094), which are also linked to type 2 diabetes (Pierce et al., 2011; Prizment et al., 2012).

1.18 Common Risk Factors

1.18.1 Obesity

Obesity and type 2 diabetes are common among those who are overweight or prediabetic (American, 2021). A comprehensive cohort study, tracking 900,000 participants for 16 years, revealed a substantially increased mortality rate from liver, pancreatic, non-Hodgkin's lymphoma, colorectal, kidney, esophageal, and multiple myeloma cancers in those with severe obesity. Cancers of the liver, colon, and rectum, as well as pancreatic, had the most impacts (Calle et al., 2003). Individuals undergoing bariatric surgery exhibited a significantly reduced occurrence of obesity-related cancers compared to severely obese control subjects (Adams et al., 2009) and also required less cancer-related medical intervention (Christou et al., 2008).

Obesity may complicate and modify the cancer-type 2 diabetes relationship. (Suh & Kim, 2019). Obesity was linked to a higher risk of cancer, most likely through mechanisms involving hormone balance, inflammation, and cellular proliferation (Byers & Sedjo, 2015), which have also been hypothesized to interact with type 2 diabetes. In a study investigating pancreatic ductal pathology, Butler and colleagues found that obese individuals without diabetes exhibited a tenfold increase in pancreatic duct replication compared to lean individuals without diabetes. Furthermore, lean individuals with diabetes showed a fourfold higher rate of duct epithelial replication compared to lean individuals without diabetes. Pancreatic exocrine neoplasia risk factors may include obesity and diabetes, according to these findings (Butler et al., 2010).

1.18.2 Hyperglycemia

Epidemiological research indicates a correlation between hyperglycemia and a higher occurrence of gastric, lung, colorectal, pancreatic, and liver cancers (de Beer & Liebenberg, 2014; Xu et al., 2016). A phenomenon known as "the Warburg effect" helps to explain cancer is encouraged by hyperglycemia (Warburg, 1956). While cancer cells typically adopt a less effective glycolytic pathway for proliferation, normal cells rely on mitochondrial oxidative phosphorylation to power cellular functions (Warburg, 1956; Vander Heiden et al., 2009). Therefore, to meet their needs for growth, cancer cells need to absorb more glucose in order to produce more energy (Devic, 2016). An imbalance in the signal transduction pathways that regulate the use of fuels and nutrients may be the cause of the cancer risk linked to diabetes (Pollak, 2008).

Advanced glycation end products (AGEs) are produced in response to hyperglycemia. By activating NF-κB and producing ROS in cells, AGEs frequently interact with their particular receptor, RAGE, speeding up oxidative stress, which in turn increases pro-inflammatory signaling (Abe & Yamagishi, 2008). Studies suggest that epithelial cell tumor transformation is aided by AGE pathway activation (Vander Heiden et al., 2009). Clinical trials have also shown a favorable connection among the AGE/RAGE interaction and the occurrence of gastric cancer (Sparvero et al., 2009), pancreatic cancer (Kuniyasu et al., 2002), and melanoma (Takada et al., 2004). Hyperglycemia promotes the proliferation of pancreatic cancer cells, according to Han et al. (Abe et al., 2004), because it activates the EGF receptor and induces the synthesis of epithelial growth factor (EGF). Furthermore, structural lung damage may be induced by hyperglycemia, which has been linked to lung cancer (Han et al., 2011). Furthermore, high glucose levels have been shown to initiate carcinogenesis by causing DNA damage (Lee et al., 2009).

1.18.3 Hyperinsulinemia

Hyperinsulinemia has been linked to an increased risk of many cancers, according to epidemiological research (Calle & Kaaks, 2004; Stolzenberg-Solomon et al.,

2005). These cancers include breast, pancreatic, ovarian, colon, renal ones, and endometrial. Additionally, insulin and the insulin receptor (IR) have been shown to play a major role in cancer biology in both in vitro and in vivo studies (Friberg et al., 2007). The growth hormone receptor (GHR) was upregulated, and GHR signaling was enhanced under hyperinsulinemic conditions, which led to an increase in hepatic IGF-1 synthesis (Frasca et al., 2008).

There is evidence from epidemiological studies and meta-analyses that higher IGF-1 levels are associated with an increased risk of cancers such as colorectal lung, prostate, and premenopausal breast (Baxter et al., 1980). IGF-1 treatment boosted the growth of cancer cells and their ability to spread to other locations, according to research on animals. Conversely, the tumor's growth was suppressed when the Igf-1 gene was knocked out (Chen et al., 2009). Furthermore, in mice models, the development of colon cancer has also been linked to IGF-2 overexpression (Yakar et al., 2005). The PI3K/Akt/mTOR signaling pathway, when activated by insulin, IGF-1, and IGF-2, may contribute to the progression of cancer (Sakatani et al., 2005; Gallagher & LeRoith, 2010).

2 Lifestyle Choices: Fueling the Flames or Extinguishing Them

Obesity, smoking, advancing age, lack of physical exercise, and unhealthy eating habits are some of the risk factors for both diabetes and cancer (Carlberg & Muñoz, 2022). The adoption of a Westernized lifestyle has led to a significant increase in obesity, which, along with conditions like hyperinsulinemia, hyperglycemia, and an inflammatory cytokine milieu (TNF-α, IL-6, IL-17, and TGF-β), plays a crucial role in the development of both type 2 diabetes (T2D) and cancer (Ferlay et al., 2019; Vella et al., 2018). Adipose tissue homeostasis is disturbed by excess body weight, leading to the secretion of inflammatory cytokines including TNF-α and IL-6. These cytokines boost cell proliferation, damage DNA, promote point mutations, angiogenesis, and tumor cell invasiveness, all of which are crucial to cancer formation (Lazarus & Bays, 2022).

According to the Diabetes Prevention Program (DPP), whereas metformin medication only lowered C-reactive protein (CRP) by 13%, weight loss resulted in a 31% decrease in CRP levels (Haffner et al., 2005). This suggests that by reducing inflammation, lifestyle changes alone—without the use of medication therapy—can successfully lower insulin resistance, slow the progression of prediabetes to type 2 diabetes, and minimize the occurrence of problems related to diabetes.

Another important component is physical activity. Increased exercise has been demonstrated to cut cancer risk by 10–25%, and research indicates that it also lowers the incidence of a number of malignancies, such as colorectal, bladder, and breast cancer (Mctiernan et al., 2019; Clemente-Suárez et al., 2023). On the other hand, adipose tissue fat buildup from physical inactivity triggers inflammatory pathways that aid in the formation of tumors (Wang & Zhou, 2021).

Smoking and alcohol use are other major causes of cancer development. Drinking alcohol damages genetic material and encourages the development of tumors by causing oxidative stress and inflammation. This is analogous to how smoking increases the risk of cancer by triggering the production of reactive oxygen and nitrogen species in the body. These species may lead to oxidative stress over time and damage proteins, lipids, and DNA (Caliri et al., 2021; Münzel et al., 2020). Crucially, antidiabetic medications that also have anti-inflammatory properties, when paired with lifestyle changes, offer a dual advantage by lowering the risk of diabetes and cancer (Olatunde et al., 2021). These treatments enhance general metabolic health in addition to halting the advancement of the disease.

3 Therapeutic Implications

3.1 Targeting Inflammation: Novel Anti-inflammatory Strategies

Hyperglycemia plays a key role in the synthesis of AGEs, which in turn increase inflammation and the generation of ROS, two molecules that have been linked to cancer progression (Ceriello et al., 2009; Huang et al., 2014). One feature of cancer development is the increased resistance to oxidative stress that epithelial cells develop as a result of prolonged activation of the AGE pathway (Yang et al., 2015; Li et al., 2017). Furthermore, AGEs fuel the inflammatory milieu inside tumors, intensifying cancer and increasing the likelihood of metastasis (Zhang et al., 2018).

It has been demonstrated that antidiabetic medications, including thiazolidinediones, biguanides, and sulfonylureas, inhibit these pathways, offering therapeutic advantages in the setting of diabetes and cancer. These medications aid in controlling hyperglycemia, lowering hyperinsulinemia, and reducing obesity, oxidative stress, and inflammation—all of which are important metabolic variables that connect diabetes to cancer (Olatunde et al., 2021; Agrawal & Kant, 2014). For instance, the biguanide metformin has shown anticancer effects, most likely by lowering insulin levels, promoting apoptosis, and inhibiting the growth of cancer cells (Evans et al., 2005; Alimova et al., 2015).

Since they not only lessen systemic inflammation but also cause cancer cells to undergo apoptosis by altering proteins involved in programmed cell death, anti-inflammatory drugs are essential in cancer treatment (Evans et al., 2005). The anti-inflammatory effects of PPARγ, which inhibits the production of cytokines such prostaglandin E2 (PGE2), TNF-α, IL-6, and IL-1β, have been shown in several studies (Alimova et al., 2015). This inhibition reduces the chronic inflammatory milieu, which is one of the key drivers of cancer's genesis and spread.

Furthermore, by blocking matrix metalloproteinases and vascular endothelial growth factor, two substances implicated in tumor angiogenesis and disruption of the blood-brain barrier, selective cyclooxygenase-2 (COX-2) inhibitors and corticosteroids such as dexamethasone, have demonstrated effectiveness in lowering neurotoxicity (Ponthan et al., 2007). By stabilizing the blood-brain barrier, these medications prevent tumor cells from invading the brain. By showing that extensive lifestyle treatments led to a 31% decrease in C-reactive protein (CRP) levels, a measure of inflammation, the Diabetes Prevention Program (DPP) study brought attention to the significance of lifestyle changes (Haffner et al., 2005). These results highlight how important lifestyle choices like nutrition and exercise are in lowering the inflammatory burden linked to cancer and diabetes.

Furthermore, the increasing amount of data demonstrating how physical activity lowers the risk of cancer further supports the link between cancer prevention and metabolic health. In addition to enhancing glucose metabolism, exercise also lowers systemic inflammation, which promotes the spread of cancer (Mctiernan et al., 2019; Clemente-Suárez et al., 2023).

3.2 Antioxidant Therapies: Boosting the Body's Defenses

Increased amounts of free radicals and a weakened antioxidant defense system are linked to diabetes, especially when it is not properly managed. These elements play a major role in oxidative stress, which is associated with DNA damage and other cellular dysfunctions that raise the chance of developing cancer. Oxidative stress, in diabetes, is not merely a consequence of hyperglycemia; it actively participates in the core mechanisms that drive cancer development. Hyperglycemia (high blood sugar) and hyperinsulinemia (high insulin) can cause cell damage responses like oxidative stress, lipotoxicity, and glucotoxicity, which can turn healthy cells into cancerous ones and raise the risk of cancer development (Han et al., 2017; Candelario-Jalil et al., 2007).

One of the initial stages of carcinogenesis is DNA damage brought on by oxidative stress, which is fueled by high glucose levels. The possibility of malignant cell transformation is increased by the ways in which this damage appears, including transcriptional pause, replication mistakes, and genomic instability (Haffner et al., 2005). Oxidative stress and chronic hyperglycemia can promote cancer growth and metastasis. Extensive research studies have demonstrated a correlation between oxidative damage and elevated glucose levels, with diabetes being associated with an elevated risk of developing various cancers, such as pancreatic, liver, and breast cancers (Aggarwal et al., 2012; Verma et al., 2017).

This issue is compounded by the strong association between oxidative stress and chronic inflammation, a known contributor to cancer risk. The persistent low-level inflammation observed in both diabetes and oxidative stress can modulate the expression of key genes and interfere with signaling cascades essential for cell survival, growth, and programmed cell death. These pathways, which include the NF-kB and MAP-kinase/AP-1 pathways, are essential for controlling cellular functions that, when disrupted, might result in unchecked cell proliferation and the development of tumors (Holcomb et al., 2015). It is significant to note that NF-kB exhibits hyperactivation in various cancer types, including breast cancer, pancreatic cancer, and hematological malignancies (Brown et al., 2015; Kato et al., 2015).

Although antioxidant treatments, such alpha-lipoic acid and DPP-4 inhibitors, are frequently used to treat diabetes and have shown promise in lowering oxidative stress, their relationship to cancer is still up for debate. According to certain research, these antioxidants may unintentionally encourage cancer spread in animal models, even though they are helpful in reducing the negative consequences of oxidative stress in diabetes (Zhou et al., 2019). The potential for antioxidants to promote tumor growth rather than stop it underscores the difficulty of applying such treatments in the context of cancer prevention, even though the exact mechanisms underlying this are not entirely understood.

3.3 Personalized Medicine: Tailoring Treatments to Individual Needs

By reducing blood glucose levels, SGLT-2 inhibitors, including canagliflozin and dapagliflozin, are frequently used to treat type 2 diabetes (T2D). They increase the excretion of glucose in the urine by blocking the sodium-glucose cotransporter 2 (SGLT2) in the kidneys, which decreases glucose reabsorption. The potential benefits of SGLT-2 inhibitors in cancer prevention and therapy are being further explored, in addition to their role in lowering blood sugar. It is worth noting that SGLT2 expression is higher in some cancers, including pancreatic and prostate tumors (Kato et al., 2015). This implies that SGLT2 inhibitors might provide a distinct treatment approach for both diabetes control and cancer prevention, particularly in malignancies where SGLT2 overexpression is present. Furthermore, preliminary studies have suggested that SGLT2 inhibitors may have anticancer effects; nevertheless, more studies in humans with cancer patients are needed to draw firm conclusions about their efficacy (Zhou et al., 2019).

Metformin, initial treatment for type 2 diabetes, primarily reduces blood glucose and insulin requirements by suppressing glucose production in the liver. By lowering hyperglycemia, it may lower the risk of cancer and improve prognosis. While primarily known for its role in diabetes therapy, metformin has been shown to lower cancer risk and enhance cancer patients' prognosis.

Multiple observational studies suggest a protective effect of metformin against various malignancies, including liver, colorectal, and breast cancer (Evans et al., 2005). This is supported by a meta-analysis, which found a substantial reduction in cancer risk among diabetic individuals taking metformin (Zhang et al., 2014). Preclinical studies, including a mouse model of lung cancer, have shown that metformin treatment significantly suppresses neoplastic cell proliferation (Alimova et al., 2015). These results provide credence to the theory that metformin's potential as an anticancer drug may be largely dependent on its effects on insulin sensitivity and glucose metabolism.

Acarbose, along with other alpha-glucosidase inhibitors like voglibose and miglitol, is commonly prescribed for type 2 diabetes due to its ability to delay carbohydrate digestion and absorption, thereby controlling postprandial blood glucose. Studies suggest these agents may also modulate the gut microbiome, potentially influencing intestinal cell proliferation and, consequently, cancer risk. Acarbose may lower the incidence of colorectal cancer by changing the composition of the gut microbiota and lowering systemic inflammation, according to a study. These results highlight the need for more investigation into alpha-glucosidase inhibitors' potential to prevent cancer, especially gastrointestinal cancers (Nagata et al., 2017).

PPARγ agonists known as thiazolidinediones (TZDs), which include pioglitazone and rosiglitazone, increase insulin sensitivity and decrease blood sugar and cholesterol levels. Despite the established advantages of thiazolidinediones (TZDs) in type 2 diabetes treatment, the study of their possible effects on cancer risk is ongoing. Meta-analyses have indicated that TZDs may offer a protective effect against some cancers, including colorectal and breast cancer (Kang et al., 2013; Wang et al., 2018). However, worries about weight gain and cardiovascular risk have hampered their use. TZDs may still be helpful in preventing cancer in spite of these worries, especially in cases where the disease is impacted by the insulin and glucose metabolism pathways.

However, several studies have linked long-acting insulin analogs, such glargine, to an increased risk of cancer. Although insulin is an essential hormone for controlling blood sugar, its mitogenic qualities, especially when taken in excess, have sparked worries about how it can encourage cell division and enhance the risk of cancer. According to a different study, patients who took long-acting insulin analogs were more likely than those who took shorter-acting insulin forms to develop some types of cancer, including breast cancer. As a result, the use of long-acting insulin in diabetes patients who are at risk for cancer is now being closely examined (Jørgensen et al., 2012).

Although its processes are different from those of other diabetes drugs, canagliflozin, a particular SGLT-2 inhibitor, has demonstrated promise in preventing the growth of cancer. Canagliflozin, in contrast to dapagliflozin, inhibits cancer progression by reducing complex I of the mitochondrial respiratory chain, an essential step in cellular energy generation and proliferation, in a way that is not AMPK-dependent (Miller et al., 2017). Beyond its function in glucose regulation, canagliflozin may have special anticancer qualities according to this novel mechanism of action; nevertheless, further study is required to fully investigate this possibility in clinical settings.

4 Conclusion

4.1 Breaking the Cycle: Preventing and Managing Diabetes and Cancer

Diabetes and cancer have a complicated association because they share risk factors such metabolic dysregulation, oxidative stress, and chronic inflammation. Managing one can have an impact on the other, as the two conditions frequently coexist. An integrated strategy that addresses these common mechanisms—reducing inflammation, enhancing metabolic regulation, and addressing oxidative stress—is necessary for the prevention and management of these disorders. The loop of diabetes to cancer advancement may be broken with the use of strategies that treat both conditions at the same time. Studies suggest that blood glucose-regulating medications, such as metformin, may also lower the risk of cancer, and lifestyle changes that reduce obesity and enhance insulin sensitivity may also be beneficial (Alimova et al., 2015; Sears et al., 2016).

4.2 The Future of Research: Unlocking New Therapeutic Targets

Finding novel therapeutic targets that can treat cancer and diabetes is the key to the future of research. Personalized treatment plans that maximize glucose control and reduce the risk of cancer may become possible because of developments in precision medicine, genomics, and biomarker discovery. A better knowledge of the environmental and genetic factors that cause these disorders will allow for the creation of more effective therapies. Furthermore, treatments that focus on common metabolic pathways, like mitochondrial function and glycolysis, are showing promise in the treatment of both disorders (Zhou et al., 2019; Matsui et al., 2015). Investigating the function of immunotherapies and the microbiota opens up new possibilities for ending the diabetes-cancer cycle. To comprehend the long-term ramifications of diabetes treatments and to create safer substitutes that do not raise the likelihood of cancer, nonetheless, a great deal more investigation is required (Evans et al., 2005; Giovannucci et al., 2016).

In conclusion, there is great potential for managing diabetes and preventing cancer with the development of personalized medicine, which involves customizing medicines for each patient based on genetic, metabolic, and lifestyle characteristics. The interaction between cancer risk and diabetic treatments highlights the need for more study to find medications that can safely treat both disorders. In addition to their use in the treatment of diabetes, medications such as SGLT-2 inhibitors, metformin, and TZDs may prove to be effective weapons in the fight against cancer as our understanding of the molecular pathways behind these conditions advances.

References

Abe, R., Shimizu, T., Sugawara, H., Watanabe, H., Nakamura, H., Choei, H., et al. (2004). Regulation of human melanoma growth and metastasis by AGE-AGE receptor interactions. *The Journal of Investigative Dermatology, 122*, 461–467.

Abe, R., & Yamagishi, S. (2008). AGE-RAGE system and carcinogenesis. *Current Pharmaceutical Design, 14*, 940–945.

Adams, T. D., Stroup, A. M., Gress, R. E., Adams, K. F., Calle, E. E., Smith, S. C., et al. (2009). Cancer incidence and mortality after gastric bypass surgery. *Obesity, 17*, 796–802.

Aggarwal, B. B., Vijayalekshmi, R. V., & Sung, B. (2009). Targeting inflammatory pathways for prevention and therapy of cancer: Short-term friend, long-term foe. *Clinical Cancer Research, 15*, 425–430.

Aggarwal, B. B., et al. (2012). Inflammation and cancer: How inflammation influences cancer development. *Clinical Cancer Research.*
Aggeli, I. K., Theofilatos, D., Beis, I., & Gaitanaki, C. (2011). Insulin-induced oxidative stress up-regulates heme oxygenase-1 via diverse signaling cascades in the C2 skeletal myoblast cell line. *Endocrinology, 152*, 1274–1283.
Agrawal, N. K., & Kant, S. (2014). Targeting inflammation in diabetes: Newer therapeutic options. *World Journal of Diabetes, 5*(5), 697–710.
Alimova, I. N., et al. (2015). Metformin as a cancer preventive agent: Mechanisms of action. *Oncology Reports.*
Ambade, A., & Mandrekar, P. (2012). Oxidative stress and inflammation: Essential partners in alcoholic liver disease. *International Journal of Hepatology, 2012*, 853175.
Amelio, I., Cutruzzolá, F., Antonov, A., Agostini, M., & Melino, G. (2014). Serine and glycine metabolism in cancer. *Trends in Biochemical Sciences, 39*, 191–198.
Amelio, I., Inoue, S., Markert, E. K., Levine, A. J., Knight, R. A., Mak, T. W., & Melino, G. (2015). TAp73 opposes tumor angiogenesis by promoting hypoxia-inducible factor 1α degradation. *Proceedings of the National Academy of Sciences of the United States of America, 112*, 226–231.
Amelio, I., & Melino, G. (2015). The p53 family and the hypoxia-inducible factors (HIFs): Determinants of cancer progression. *Trends in Biochemical Sciences, 40*, 425–434.
American, D. A. (2021). 2. Classification and diagnosis of diabetes: Standards of medical care in diabetes-2021. *Diabetes Care, 44*, S15–S33.
Asiri, A., Al Qarni, A., & Bakillah, A. (2024). The interlinking metabolic association between type 2 diabetes mellitus and cancer: Molecular mechanisms and therapeutic insights. *Diagnostics, 14*(19), 2132.
Azoury, S. C., et al. (2015). Immune checkpoint inhibitors for cancer therapy: Clinical efficacy and safety. *Current Cancer Drug Targets, 15*(6), 452–462.
Balkwill, F., & Mantovani, A. (2001). Inflammation and cancer: Back to Virchow? *Lancet, 357*, 539–545.
Barroso-Sousa, R., et al. (2018). Incidence of endocrine dysfunction following the use of different immune checkpoint inhibitor regimens: A systematic review and meta-analysis. *JAMA Oncology, 4*(2), 173–182.
Baxter, R. C., Bryson, J. M., & Turtle, J. R. (1980). Somatogenic receptors of rat liver: Regulation by insulin. *Endocrinology, 107*, 1176–1181.
Bjornsdottir, H. H., Rawshani, A., Rawshani, A., Franzén, S., Svensson, A.-M., Sattar, N., & Gudbjörnsdottir, S. (2020). A national observation study of cancer incidence and mortality risks in type 2 diabetes compared to the background population over time. *Scientific Reports, 10*, 1–12.
Brown, M. D., et al. (2015). The potential risks of antioxidants in cancer therapy. *Journal of Cancer Therapy.*
Butler, A. E., Galasso, R., Matveyenko, A., Rizza, R. A., Dry, S., & Butler, P. C. (2010). Pancreatic duct replication is increased with obesity and type 2 diabetes in humans. *Diabetologia, 53*, 21–26.
Byers, T., & Sedjo, R. L. (2015). Body fatness as a cause of cancer: Epidemiologic clues to biologic mechanisms. *Endocrine-Related Cancer, 22*, R125–R134.
Byun, D. J., et al. (2017). Cancer immunotherapy - immune checkpoint blockade and associated endocrinopathies. *Nature Reviews. Endocrinology, 13*(4), 195–207.
Caliri, A. W., Tommasi, S., & Besaratinia, A. (2021). Relationships among smoking, oxidative stress, inflammation, macromolecular damage, and cancer. *Mutation Research, Reviews in Mutation Research, 787*, 108365.
Calle, E. E., & Kaaks, R. (2004). Overweight, obesity and cancer: Epidemiological evidence and proposed mechanisms. *Nature Reviews. Cancer, 4*(8), 579–591.
Calle, E. E., Rodriguez, C., Walker-Thurmond, K., & Thun, M. J. (2003). Overweight, obesity, and mortality from cancer in a prospectively studied cohort of U.S. adults. *New England Journal of Medicine, 348*, 1625–1638.

Candelario-Jalil, E., et al. (2007). Cyclooxygenase inhibition limits blood-brain barrier disruption following intracerebral injection of tumor necrosis factor-α in the rat. *The Journal of Pharmacology and Experimental Therapeutics, 323*, 488–498.

Carlberg, C., & Muñoz, A. (2022). An update on vitamin D signaling and cancer. In *Seminars in cancer biology*. Elsevier.

Centers for Disease Control and Prevention. (2020). *About "NIOSH"*.

Ceriello, A., et al. (2009). Oxidative stress and diabetes: The possible role of antioxidants. *Journal of Clinical & Translational Endocrinology*.

Chan, K. K., & Bass, A. R. (2020). Autoimmune complications of immunotherapy: Pathophysiology and management. *BMJ (Clinical research ed.), 369*, m736.

Chen, W., Wang, S., Tian, T., Bai, J., Hu, Z., Xu, Y., et al. (2009). Phenotypes and genotypes of insulin-like growth factor 1, IGF-binding protein-3 and cancer risk: Evidence from 96 studies. *European Journal of Human Genetics, 17*, 1668–1675.

Cho, J., Seo, J., Lim, C. H., Yang, L., Shiratsuchi, T., Lee, M.-H., Chowdhury, R. R., Kasahara, H., Kim, J.-S., Oh, S. P., Lee, Y. J., & Terada, N. (2015). Mitochondrial ATP transporter Ant2 depletion impairs erythropoiesis and B lymphopoiesis. *Cell Death and Differentiation, 22*, 1437–1450.

Christou, N. V., Lieberman, M., Sampalis, F., & Sampalis, J. S. (2008). Bariatric surgery reduces cancer risk in morbidly obese patients. *Surgery for Obesity and Related Diseases, 4*, 691–695.

Cignarelli, A., Genchi, V. A., Caruso, I., Natalicchio, A., Perrini, S., Laviola, L., et al. (2018). Diabetes and cancer: Pathophysiological fundamentals of a 'dangerous affair'. *Diabetes Research and Clinical Practice, 143*, 378–388.

Clemente-Suárez, V. J., Martín-Rodríguez, A., Redondo-Flórez, L., Ruisoto, P., Navarro-Jiménez, E., Ramos-Campo, D. J., & Tornero-Aguilera, J. F. (2023). Metabolic health, mitochondrial fitness, physical activity, and cancer. *Cancers, 15*, 814.

Clore, J. N., & Thurby-Hay, L. (2009). Glucocorticoid-induced hyperglycemia. *Endocrine Practice, 15*, 469–474.

Coughlin, S. S., Calle, E. E., Teras, L. R., Petrelli, J., & Thun, M. J. (2004). Diabetes mellitus as a predictor of cancer mortality in a large cohort of US adults. *American Journal of Epidemiology, 159*, 1160–1167.

Coussens, L. M., & Werb, Z. (2002). Inflammation and cancer. *Nature, 420*, 860–867.

Dalla Vestra, M., Mussap, M., Gallina, P., Bruseghin, M., Cernigoi, A. M., Saller, A., Plebani, M., & Fioretto, P. (2005). Acute-phase markers of inflammation and glomerular structure in patients with type-2 diabetes. *Journal of the American Society of Nephrology, 16*, S78–S82.

de Beer, J. C., & Liebenberg, L. (2014). Does cancer risk increase with HbA1c, independent of diabetes? *British Journal of Cancer, 110*, 2361–2368.

De Velasco, G., et al. (2017). Comprehensive meta-analysis of key immune-related adverse events from CTLA-4 and PD-1/PD-L1 inhibitors in cancer patients. *Cancer Immunology Research, 5*(4), 312–318.

Devic, S. (2016). Warburg effect - A consequence or the cause of carcinogenesis? *Journal of Cancer, 7*, 817–822.

Dinarello, C. A., Donath, M. Y., & Mandrup-Poulsen, T. (2010). Role of Il-1 beta in type 2 diabetes. *Current Opinion in Endocrinology, Diabetes, and Obesity, 17*, 314–321.

Donath, M. Y., Dalmas, É., Sauter, N. S., & Böni Schnetzler, M. (2013). Inflammation in obesity and diabetes: Islet dysfunction and therapeutic opportunity. *Cell Metabolism, 17*, 860–872.

Duncan, B. B. (2017). The burden of diabetes and hyperglycaemia in Brazil: Past and present. Findings from the global burden of disease study 2015. *Diabetology & Metabolic Syndrome, 9*, 1–18.

Durackova, Z. (2009). Some current insights into oxidative stress. *Physiological Research*.

Emmendoerffer, A., Hecht, M., Boeker, T., Mueller, M., & Heinrich, U. (2000). Role of inflammation in chemical-induced lung cancer. *Toxicology Letters, 112-113*, 185–191.

Evans, J. M. M., et al. (2005). Metformin and cancer risk in patients with type 2 diabetes: A systematic review. *Diabetes Care*.

Fatima, M. T., Islam, Z., Ahmad, E., & Salahuddin, P. (2018). Emerging targets and latest proteomics based therapeutic approaches in neurodegenerative diseases. *Current Protein & Peptide Science, 19*, 858–875.

Ferlay, J., Colombet, M., Soerjomataram, I., Mathers, C., Parkin, D. M., Piñeros, M., et al. (2019). Estimating the global cancer incidence and mortality in 2018: GLOBOCAN sources and methods. *International Journal of Cancer, 144*, 1941–1953.

Fialkow, L., Wang, Y., & Downey, G. P. (2007). Reactive oxygen and nitrogen species as signaling molecules regulating neutrophil function. *Free Radical Biology & Medicine, 42*, 153–164.

Frasca, F., Pandini, G., Sciacca, L., Pezzino, V., Squatrito, S., Belfiore, A., et al. (2008). The role of insulin receptors and IGF-I receptors in cancer and other diseases. *Archives of Physiology and Biochemistry, 114*, 23–37.

Friberg, E., Mantzoros, C. S., & Wolk, A. (2007). Diabetes and risk of endometrial cancer: A population-based prospective cohort study. *Cancer Epidemiology, Biomarkers & Prevention, 16*, 276–280.

Fridovich, I. (1978). The biology of oxygen radicals. *Science, 201*, 875–880.

Gallagher, E. J., & LeRoith, D. (2010). The proliferating role of insulin and insulin-like growth factors in cancer. *Trends in Endocrinology and Metabolism, 21*, 610–618.

Giovannucci, E., et al. (2016). Insulin and cancer: Exploring the link between insulin analogues and cancer risk. *Cancer Epidemiology.*

González, P., Lozano, P., Ros, G., & Solano, F. (2023). Hyperglycemia and oxidative stress: An integral, updated and critical overview of their metabolic interconnections. *International Journal of Molecular Sciences, 24*, 9352.

Goossens, V., De Vos, K., Vercammen, D., Steemans, M., Vancompernolle, K., Fiers, W., Vandenabeele, P., & Grooten, J. (1999). Redox regulation of TNF signaling. *BioFactors, 10*, 145–156.

Goossens, V., Grooten, J., De Vos, K., & Fiers, W. (1995). Direct evidence for tumor necrosis factor-induced mitochondrial reactive oxygen intermediates and their involvement in cytotoxicity. *Proceedings of the National Academy of Sciences of the United States of America, 92*, 8115–8119.

Grivennikov, S. I., Greten, F. R., & Karin, M. (2010). Immunity, inflammation, and cancer. *Cell, 140*, 883–899.

Gumieniczek, A., Hopkała, H., Roliński, J., & Bojarska-Junak, A. (2005). Antioxidative and anti-inflammatory effects of repaglinide in plasma of diabetic animals. *Pharmacological Research, 52*, 162–166.

Haffner, S., Temprosa, M., Crandall, J., Fowler, S., Goldberg, R., Horton, E., Marcovina, S., Mather, K., Orchard, T., Ratner, R., et al. (2005). Intensive lifestyle intervention or metformin on inflammation and coagulation in participants with impaired glucose tolerance. *Diabetes, 54*, 1566–1572.

Han, L., Ma, Q., Li, J., Liu, H., Li, W., Ma, G., et al. (2011). High glucose promotes pancreatic cancer cell proliferation via the induction of EGF expression and transactivation of EGFR. *PLoS One, 6*, e27074.

Han, Q., Yuan, Q., & Xie, G. (2017). 6-Shogaol attenuates LPS-induced inflammation in BV2 microglia cells by activating PPAR-γ. *Oncotarget, 8*(26), 42001–42006.

Harcourt, B. E., Penfold, S. A., & Forbes, J. M. (2013). Coming full circle in diabetes mellitus: From complications to initiation. *Nature Reviews Endocrinology, 9*(2), 113–123.

Holcomb, I., et al. (2015). NF-kB as a target for cancer therapy. *Current Oncology Reports.*

Hold, G. L., & El-Omar, E. M. (2008). Genetic aspects of inflammation and cancer. *The Biochemical Journal, 410*, 225–235.

Hotamisligil, G. S., Shargill, N. S., & Spiegelman, B. M. (1993). Adipose expression of tumor necrosis actor- alpha: Direct role in obesity-linked insulin resistance. *Science, 259*(5091), 87–91.

Huang, X., et al. (2014). Oxidative stress in diabetes mellitus and the potential role of antioxidants in reducing cancer risk. *Endocrine Reviews.*

Hughes, J., Vudattu, N., Sznol, M., Gettinger, S., Kluger, H., Lupsa, B., & Herold, K. C. (2015). Precipitation of autoimmune diabetes with anti-PD-1 immunotherapy. *Diabetes Care, 38*, e55–e57.

Hussain, S. P., Hofseth, L. J., & Harris, C. C. (2003). Radical causes of cancer. *Nature Reviews. Cancer, 3*, 276–285.

Jabs, T. (1999). Reactive oxygen intermediates as mediators of programmed cell death in plants and animals. *Biochemical Pharmacology, 57*, 231–245.

Jesmin, J., Rashid, M. S., Jamil, H., Hontecillas, R., & Bassaganya-Riera, J. (2010). Gene regulatory network reveals oxidative stress as the underlying molecular mechanism of type 2 diabetes and hypertension. *BMC Medical Genomics, 3*, 45.

Jørgensen, M. E., et al. (2012). Insulin glargine and cancer risk: A cohort study of patients with type 2 diabetes. *Diabetes Care.*

Joussen, A. M., Poulaki, V., Mitsiades, N., Kirchhof, B., Koizumi, K., Döhmen, S., & Adamis, A. P. (2002). Non-steroidal anti-inflammatory drugs prevent early diabetic retinopathy via TNF-alpha suppression. *The FASEB Journal, 16*, 438–440.

Kang, J. H., et al. (2013). Thiazolidinediones and cancer risk: A systematic review and meta-analysis. *Diabetes, Obesity and Metabolism.*

Kato, M., et al. (2015). Expression of SGLT2 in cancer cells: Implications for cancer therapy. *Oncotarget.*

Khalid, M., Petroianu, G., & Adem, A. (2022). Advanced glycation end products and diabetes mellitus: Mechanisms and perspectives. *Biomolecules, 12*, 542.

Klein, A. P. (2012). Genetic susceptibility to pancreatic cancer. *Molecular Carcinogenesis, 51*, 14–24.

Kuniyasu, H., Oue, N., Wakikawa, A., Shigeishi, H., Matsutani, N., Kuraoka, K., et al. (2002). Expression of receptors for advanced glycation end-products (RAGE) is closely associated with the invasive and metastatic activity of gastric cancer. *The Journal of Pathology, 196*, 163–170.

Lazarus, E., & Bays, H. E. (2022). Cancer and obesity: An obesity medicine association (OMA) clinical practice statement (CPS) 2022. *Obesity Pillars, 3*, 100026.

Lee, G., Walser, T. C., & Dubinett, S. M. (2009). Chronic inflammation, chronic obstructive pulmonary disease, and lung cancer. *Current Opinion in Pulmonary Medicine, 15*, 303–307.

Li, C., et al. (2017). Diabetes and cancer: A review of the mechanisms linking hyperglycemia and tumor progression. *Cancer Research and Treatment.*

Lin, W. W., & Karin, M. (2007). A cytokine-mediated link between innate immunity, inflammation, and cancer. *The Journal of Clinical Investigation, 117*, 1175–1183.

Ling, S., Brown, K., Miksza, J. K., Howells, L., Morrison, A., Issa, E., Yates, T., Khunti, K., Davies, M. J., & Zaccardi, F. (2020). Association of type 2 diabetes with cancer: A meta-analysis with bias analysis for unmeasured confounding in 151 cohorts comprising 32 million people. *Diabetes Care, 43*, 2313–2322.

Liu, J., Ren, Z. H., Qiang, H., Wu, J., Shen, M., Zhang, L., & Lyu, J. (2020). Trends in the incidence of diabetes mellitus: Results from the Global Burden of Disease Study 2017 and implications for diabetes mellitus prevention. *BMC Public Health, 20*, 1415.

Liu, X., Ji, J., Sundquist, K., Sundquist, J., & Hemminki, K. (2012). The impact of type 2 diabetes mellitus on cancer-specific survival: A follow-up study in Sweden. *Cancer, 118*, 1353–1361.

Livingstone, S. J., Levin, D., Looker, H. C., Lindsay, R. S., Wild, S. H., Joss, N., et al. (2015). Estimated life expectancy in a Scottish cohort with type 1 diabetes, 2008-2010. *JAMA, 313*, 37–44.

Lobo, V., Patil, A., Phatak, A., & Chandra, N. (2010). Free radicals, antioxidants and functional foods: Impact on human health. *Pharmacognosy Reviews, 4*, 118–126.

Malek, M., Aghili, R., Emami, Z., & Khamseh, M. E. (2013). Risk of cancer in diabetes: The effect of metformin. *ISRN Endocrinology, 2013*, 9.

Marciniak, S. J., Yun, C. Y., Oyadomari, S., Novoa, I., Zhang, Y., Jungreis, R., Nagata, K., Harding, H. P., & Ron, D. (2004). HOP induces death by promoting protein synthesis and oxidation in the stressed endoplasmic reticulum. *Genes & Development, 18*, 3066–3077.

Matsui, T., et al. (2015). PPARγ and cancer: The role of pioglitazone in tumorigenesis. *Oncological Reviews*.

Mctiernan, A., Friedenreich, C. M., Katzmarzyk, P. T., Powell, K. E., Macko, R., Buchner, D., Pescatello, L. S., Bloodgood, B., Tennant, B., Vaux-Bjerke, A., et al. (2019). Physical activity in cancer prevention and survival: A systematic review. *Medicine and Science in Sports and Exercise, 51*, 1252.

Mei, H., Sun, S., Bai, Y., Chen, Y., Chai, R., & Li, H. (2015). Reduced mtDNA copy number increases the sensitivity of tumor cells to chemotherapeutic drugs. *Cell Death & Disease, 6*, e1710.

Miliara, X., Garnett, J. A., Tatsuta, T., Abid Ali, F., Baldie, H., Pérez-Dorado, I., Simpson, P., Yague, E., Langer, T., & Matthews, S. (2015). Intra-mitochondrial signaling: Interactions among mitoKATP, PKCε, ROS, and MPT. *EMBO Reports, 16*, 824–835.

Miller, R. A., et al. (2017). Canagliflozin inhibits cancer growth via AMPK-independent inhibition of complex I of the mitochondrial respiratory chain. *Journal of Clinical Investigation*.

Mittal, M., Siddiqui, M. R., Tran, K., Reddy, S. P., & Malik, A. B. (2014). Reactive oxygen species in inflammation and tissue injury. *Antioxidants & Redox Signaling, 20*, 1126–1167.

Morviducci, L., Rota, F., Rizza, L., Di Giacinto, P., Ramponi, S., Nardone, M., Tubili, C., Lenzi, A., Zuppi, P., & Baldelli, R. (2018). Everolimus is a new anti-cancer molecule: Metabolic side effects as lipid disorders and hyperglycemia. *Diabetes Research and Clinical Practice, 143*, 428–431.

Münzel, T., Hahad, O., Kuntic, M., Keaney, J. F., Jr., Deanfield, J. E., & Daiber, A. (2020). Effects of tobacco cigarettes, e-cigarettes, and waterpipe smoking on endothelial function and clinical outcomes. *European Heart Journal, 41*, 4057–4070.

Nagata, C., et al. (2017). Acarbose and the risk of colorectal cancer: A study on the effects of alpha-glucosidase inhibitors. *Journal of Clinical Oncology*.

Navarro, J. F., & Mora, C. (2005). Role of inflammation in diabetic complications. *Nephrology, Dialysis, Transplantation, 20*, 2601–2604.

Olatunde, A., Nigam, M., Singh, R. K., et al. (2021). Cancer and diabetes: The interlinking metabolic pathways and repurposing actions of antidiabetic drugs. *Cancer Cell International, 21*, 499.

Pardoll, D. M. (2012). The blockade of immune checkpoints in cancer immunotherapy. *Nature Reviews. Cancer, 12*(4), 252–264.

Pickup, J. C. (2004). Inflammation and activated immune system in the pathogenesis of type 2 diabetes. *Diabetes Care, 27*, 813–823.

Pierce, B. L., Austin, M. A., & Ahsan, H. (2011). Association study of type 2 diabetes genetic susceptibility variants and risk of pancreatic cancer: An analysis of PanScan-I data. *Cancer Causes & Control, 22*, 877–883.

Piro, S., Anello, M., Di Pietro, C., Lizzio, M. N., Patanè, G., Rabuazzo, A. M., Vigneri, R., Purrello, M., & Purrello, F. (2002). Chronic exposure to free fatty acids or high glucose induces apoptosis in rat pancreatic islets: Possible role of oxidative stress. *Metabolism, 51*, 1340–1347.

Płachetka, A., Adamek, B., Strzelczyk, J. K., Krakowczyk, Ł., Migula, P., Nowak, P., et al. (2013). 8-hydroxy-2′-deoxyguanosine in colorectal adenocarcinoma–is it a result of oxidative stress? *Medical Science Monitor, 19*, 690–695.

Pollak, M. (2008). Insulin and insulin-like growth factor signalling in neoplasia. *Nature Reviews. Cancer, 8*, 915–928.

Ponthan, F., et al. (2007). Celecoxib prevents neuroblastoma tumor development and potentiates the effect of chemotherapeutic drugs in vitro and in vivo. *Clinical Cancer Research, 3*, 1036–1044.

Postow, M. A., et al. (2018). Immune-related adverse events associated with immune checkpoint blockade. *The New England Journal of Medicine, 378*(2), 158–168.

Poyton, R. O., Ball, K. A., & Castello, P. R. (2009). Mitochondrial generation of free radicals and hypoxic signaling. *Trends in Endocrinology and Metabolism, 20*, 332–340.

Pradhan, A. D., Manson, J. E., Rifai, N., Buring, J. E., & Ridker, P. M. (2001). C-reactive protein, interleukin 6 and risk of developing type 2 diabetes mellitus. *JAMA, 286*, 327–334.

Prizment, A. E., Gross, M., Rasmussen-Torvik, L., Peacock, J. M., & Anderson, K. E. (2012). Genes related to diabetes may be associated with pancreatic cancer in a population-based case-control study in Minnesota. *Pancreas, 41*, 50–53.

Quandt, Z., et al. (2020). Autoimmune endocrinopathies: An emerging complication of immune checkpoint inhibitors. *Annual Review of Medicine, 72*, 313–330.

Rehman, K., & Akash, M. S. H. (2017). Mechanism of generation of oxidative stress and pathophysiology of type 2 diabetes mellitus: How are they interlinked? *Journal of Cellular Biochemistry, 118*, 3577–3585.

Ribas, A., & Wolchok, J. D. (2018). Cancer immunotherapy using checkpoint blockade. *Science, 359*(6382), 1350–1355.

Ricart, W., & Fernández-Real, J. M. (2001). No decrease in free IGF-I with increasing insulin in obesity-related insulin resistance. *Obesity Research, 9*(10), 631–636.

Rivlin, N., Brosh, R., Oren, M., & Rotter, V. (2011). Mutations in the p53 tumor suppressor gene: Important milestones at the various steps of tumorigenesis. *Genes & Cancer, 2*, 466–474.

Sainz, R. M., Lombo, F., & Mayo, J. C. (2012). Radical decisions in cancer: Redox control of cell growth and death. *Cancers (Basel), 4*, 442–474.

Sakatani, T., Kaneda, A., Iacobuzio-Donahue, C. A., Carter, M. G., de Boom Witzel, S., Okano, H., et al. (2005). Loss of imprinting of Igf2 alters intestinal maturation and tumorigenesis in mice. *Science, 307*, 1976–1978.

Santibáñez-Andrade, M., Quezada-Maldonado, E. M., Rivera-Pineda, A., Chirino, Y. I., García-Cuellar, C. M., & Sánchez-Pérez, Y. (2023). The road to malignant cell transformation after particulate matter exposure: From oxidative stress to genotoxicity. *International Journal of Molecular Sciences, 24*, 1782.

Saydah, S. H., Loria, C. M., Eberhardt, M. S., & Brancati, F. L. (2003). Abnormal glucose tolerance and the risk of cancer death in the United States. *American Journal of Epidemiology, 157*, 1092–1100.

Schetter, A. J., Heegaard, N. H., & Harris, C. C. (2010). Inflammation and cancer: Interweaving microRNA, free radical, cytokine and p53 pathways. *Carcinogenesis, 31*, 37–49.

Schmidt, M. I., Duncan, B. B., Sharrett, A. R., Lindberg, G., Savage, P. J., Offenbacher, S., Azambuja, M. I., Tracy, R. P., & Heiss, G. (1999). Markers of inflammation and prediction of diabetes mellitus in adults: A cohort study. *Lancet, 353*, 1649–1652.

Schraufstatter, I., Hyslop, P. A., Jackson, J. H., & Cochrane, C. G. (1988). Oxidant-induced DNA damage of target cells. *The Journal of Clinical Investigation, 82*, 1040–1050.

Sears, R. C., et al. (2016). Long-term risk of cancer with pioglitazone and insulin: A 20-year case-control study. *Cancer Epidemiology, Biomarkers & Prevention.*

Shahwan, M., Alhumaydhi, F., Ashraf, G. M., Hasan, P. M. Z., & Shamsi, A. (2022). Role of polyphenols in combating type 2 diabetes and insulin resistance. *International Journal of Biological Macromolecules, 206*, 567–579.

Shu, X., Ji, J., Li, X., Sundquist, J., Sundquist, K., & Hemminki, K. (2010). Cancer risk among patients hospitalized for type 1 diabetes mellitus: A population-based cohort study in Sweden. *Diabetes Medical, 27*, 791–797.

Singer, E., Judkins, J., Salomonis, N., Matlaf, L., Soteropoulos, P., McAllister, S., & Soroceanu, L. (2015). Reactive oxygen species-mediated therapeutic response and resistance in glioblastoma. *Cell Death & Disease, 6*, e1601.

Sparvero, L. J., Asafu-Adjei, D., Kang, R., Tang, D., Amin, N., Im, J., et al. (2009). RAGE (receptor for advanced glycation endproducts) and their role in cancer and inflammation. *Journal of Translational Medicine, 7*, 17.

Stamatouli, A. M., et al. (2018). Collateral damage: Insulin-dependent diabetes induced with checkpoint inhibitors. *Diabetes, 67*(8), 1471–1480.

Stevens, R. J., Roddam, A. W., & Beral, V. (2007). Pancreatic cancer in type 1 and young-onset diabetes: Systematic review and meta-analysis. *British Journal of Cancer, 96*, 507–509.

Stolzenberg-Solomon, R. Z., Graubard, B. I., Chari, S., Limburg, P., Taylor, P. R., Virtamo, J., et al. (2005). Insulin, glucose, insulin resistance, and pancreatic cancer in male smokers. *JAMA, 294*, 2872–2878.

Suh, S., & Kim, K. W. (2019). Diabetes and cancer: Cancer should be screened in routine diabetes assessment. *Diabetes and Metabolism Journal, 43*, 733–743.

Takada, M., Hirata, K., Ajiki, T., Suzuki, Y., & Kuroda, Y. (2004). Expression of receptor for advanced glycation end products (RAGE) and MMP-9 in human pancreatic cancer cells. *Hepato-Gastroenterology, 51*, 928–930.

Uceda, A. B., Mariño, L., Casasnovas, R., & Adrover, M. (2024). An overview on glycation: Molecular mechanisms, impact on proteins, pathogenesis, and inhibition. *Biophysical Reviews, 16*, 189–218.

Valko, M., Leibfritz, D., Moncol, J., Cronin, M. T., Mazur, M., & Telser, J. (2007). Free radicals and antioxidants in normal physiological functions and human disease. *The International Journal of Biochemistry & Cell Biology, 39*, 44–84.

Valko, M., Rhodes, C. J., Moncol, J., Izakovic, M., & Mazur, M. (2006). Free radicals, metals and antioxidants in oxidative stress-induced cancer. *Chemico-Biological Interactions, 160*, 1–40.

Vander Heiden, M. G., Cantley, L. C., & Thompson, C. B. (2009). Understanding the Warburg effect: The metabolic requirements of cell proliferation. *Science, 324*, 1029–1033.

Vella, V., Milluzzo, A., Scalisi, N. M., Vigneri, P., & Sciacca, L. (2018). Insulin receptor isoforms in cancer. *International Journal of Molecular Sciences, 19*, 3615.

Verma, M., et al. (2017). NF-kB activation in cancer: A potential target for novel therapeutic interventions. *Cancer Letters*.

Vikram, A., Jena, G., & Ramarao, P. (2010). Insulin-resistance and benign prostatic hyperplasia: The connection. *European Journal of Pharmacology, 641*(2–3), 75–81.

Wander, G. S., Khurana, S. B., Gulati, R., Sachar, R. K., Gupta, R. K., Khurana, S., & Anand, I. S. (1994). Epidemiology of coronary heart disease and risk factors in a rural Punjab population: Prevalence and correlation with various risk factors. *Indian Heart Journal, 46*, 319–323.

Wang, F., et al. (2018). Thiazolidinediones and cancer risk in type 2 diabetes: A meta-analysis. *PLoS One*.

Wang, Q., & Zhou, W. (2021). Roles and molecular mechanisms of physical exercise in cancer prevention and treatment. *Journal of Sport and Health Science, 10*, 201–210.

Warburg, O. (1956). On the origin of cancer cells. *Science, 123*, 309–314.

Wu, Y., & Zhou, B. P. (2010). TNF-?/NF-?B/snail pathway in cancer cell migration and invasion. *British Journal of Cancer, 102*, 639–644.

Xu, J., Ye, Y., Wu, H., Duerksen-Hughes, P., Zhang, H., Li, P., et al. (2016). Association between markers of glucose metabolism and risk of colorectal cancer. *BMJ Open, 6*, e011430.

Yadav, N., Kumar, S., Marlowe, T., Chaudhary, A. K., Kumar, R., Wang, J., O'Malley, J., Boland, P. M., Jayanthi, S., Kumar, T. K. S., Yadava, N., & Chandra, D. (2015). Oxidative phosphorylation-dependent regulation of cancer cell apoptosis in response to anticancer agents. *Cell Death & Disease, 6*, e1969.

Yakar, S., Leroith, D., & Brodt, P. (2005). The role of the growth hormone/insulin-like growth factor axis in tumor growth and progression: Lessons from animal models. *Cytokine & Growth Factor Reviews, 16*, 407–420.

Yang, Q., et al. (2015). Hyperglycemia-induced oxidative stress and cancer development in diabetes. *Journal of Diabetes Research*.

Yu, T., Robotham, J. L., & Yoon, Y. (2006). Increased production of reactive oxygen species in hyperglycemic conditions requires dynamic change of mitochondrial morphology. *Proceedings of the National Academy of Sciences of the United States of America, 103*, 2653–2658.

Zhang, M., et al. (2014). Metformin use and cancer mortality in diabetic patients: A meta-analysis. *Cancer Epidemiology, Biomarkers & Prevention*.

Zhang, Z., et al. (2018). The role of oxidative stress in diabetes-associated cancers. *Antioxidants*.

Zhao, H., Wu, L., Yan, G., Chen, Y., Zhou, M., Wu, Y., et al. (2021). Inflammation and tumor progression: Signaling pathways and targeted intervention. *Signal Transduction and Targeted Therapy, 6*, 263.

Zhou, X., et al. (2019). Potential anticancer effects of SGLT-2 inhibitors. *Diabetes & Metabolism Journal*.

Diabetes in Cancer Survivors

Mamali Das, Chandramohan Kiruthiga,
Arumugam Kamaladevi, and K. Langeswaran

Abstract

Diabetes and cancer have been known to be two frequent comorbid chronic ailments, possessing a complicated bidirectional relationship. Cancer survivors, usually referred to describe the patients who have completed primary cancer therapy and are recovering, are at higher risk of getting diabetes. Several reasons such as treatment side effects, lifestyle modification, and shared risk factors including obesity, aging, and inactivity are found to contribute to the risk. Various cancer treatment procedures like chemotherapy and hormonal therapies are found to induce β-cell dysfunction and metabolic derangements, leading to diabetes. Aside from this, there are several other factors such as weight gain and psychological distress seen in cancer survivors, which in turn enhance the risk. Contrary to this, survivors of cancer who have preexisting diabetic condition have poorer outcomes from cancer in terms of recurrence and mortality. This interaction between cancer and diabetes in two directions points toward the necessity of models that have the ability to treat both diseases in a concerted manner. The improvement of long-term health for cancer survivors calls for early detection, lifestyle intervention, and individually tailored management strategies to prevent diabetes.

Keywords

Diabetes · Cancer survivors · Insulin resistance · Metabolic syndrome · Chemotherapy · Lifestyle interventions

---

M. Das · C. Kiruthiga · A. Kamaladevi · K. Langeswaran (✉)
Department of Biomedical Science, Alagappa University, Karaikudi, Tamilnadu, India

R. Noor (ed.), *Diabetes and Cancer: Association, Mechanism, and Therapeutic Implications*, https://doi.org/10.1007/978-981-95-5651-9_4

1 Introduction

Survivorship of cancer has grown tremendously as a result of improvements in early diagnosis and treatment (DeSantis et al., 2014). Nevertheless, long-term complications such as metabolic disorders like diabetes are common among survivors. Diabetes, a chronic metabolic disorder characterized by hyperglycemia, shares several risk factors with cancer, including obesity, sedentary lifestyles, and aging. Such complications are caused by a range of factors, such as cancer therapy like radiotherapy, chemotherapy, and surgery, which may harm endocrine organs and alter hormonal balance (Chueh & Yoo, 2020a, b). For example, irradiation of the hypothalamus results in growth hormone deficiency, hypogonadism, and abnormal appetite control that leads to obesity and insulin resistance (Bizzarri et al., 2019). Moreover, chemotherapy may acutely damage beta cells of the pancreas directly with a disturbance of insulin release (Bizzarri et al., 2019). Furthermore, cancer survivorship may expose individuals to a variety of metabolic risk factors including obesity, inactivity, abnormal lipids, and insulin resistance (Gregory, 2018). Understanding the interplay between these two conditions is crucial for improving survivorship care and quality of life.

Research found two-way association between cancer and diabetes where existence of any one could increase the severity of the other. For example, cancer therapies like glucocorticoids and some chemotherapeutic drugs may cause hyperglycemia and insulin resistance and contribute to diabetes in survivors (Giovannucci et al., 2010). Moreover, survivors of cancer tend to have lifestyle modifications, including decreased physical activity and weight gain, that also contribute to metabolic dysregulation (Ligibel et al., 2019). Research has indicated that survivors of childhood cancer, especially, are more likely to develop type 2 diabetes and metabolic syndrome as a result of the long-term impact of treatments such as radiation and chemotherapy (Meacham et al., 2010). The treatment of such complications calls for multidisciplinary interventions, namely, periodic monitoring of metabolic indices, lifestyle modification, and, in certain cases, drug treatment for minimizing the risk of diabetes as well as of diabetes-related complications (Demark-Wahnefried et al., 2017). On implementing these as a part of survivorship care plans, doctors are able to largely enhance survivors' long-term health outcomes as well as improve the quality of their lives.

2 Epidemiology of Diabetes in Cancer Survivors

Cancer survivors have an increased risk of developing diabetes for several reasons, such as the metabolic effects of the cancer itself; the effects of cancer therapies like chemotherapy, radiation, and hormone therapy; and lifestyle changes after a cancer diagnosis. It is important to realize the epidemiology of diabetes among this population in order to detect diabetes early, prevent it, and manage it effectively. Figure 1 shows the epidemiology and associated risk factors of diabetes in cancer survivors.

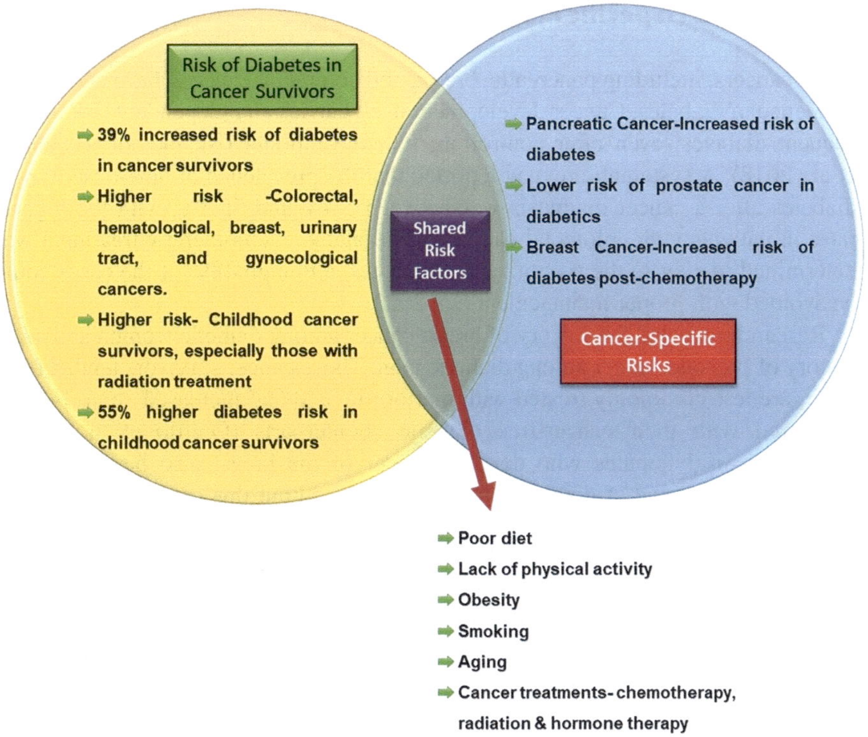

Fig. 1 Epidemiology and risk factors of diabetes in cancer survivors

2.1 Increased Risk of Diabetes in Cancer Survivors

Survivors of cancer have a higher chance of having diabetes compared to the general public. A meta-analysis of 13 cohort studies indicated that cancer survivors had a 39% elevated risk for diabetes (Xiao et al., 2021). It was most increased for survivors of colorectal, hematological, breast, urinary tract, and gynecologic cancer. Childhood cancer survivors also showed a higher risk of diabetes, with those who received total body or abdominal irradiation having the highest risk (Meacham et al., 2009).

An Ontario population-based study revealed a 55% higher rate of childhood cancer survivors with diabetes, and the survivors of leukemia and lymphoma were at higher risk (Lega et al., 2018). In addition, the correlation between cardiovascular disease and diabetes was more evident among adult cancer survivors than in the general population (Oh et al., 2023). The results highlight the need for diabetes prevention and management programs for cancer survivors.

2.2 Cancer-Specific Risk

Some cancers, including pancreatic, breast, and colorectal cancers, have a very high incidence of diabetes. Cancer development itself carries an independent risk of subsequent diabetes, even after controlling for conventional risk factors (Hwangbo et al., 2018). A systematic review reported that the prevalence of new-onset type 2 diabetes after a cancer diagnosis was between 5.4% and 55.3%, with the highest rates in patients with colorectal cancer. Additionally, chemotherapy treatment was determined to elevate the risk of type 2 diabetes, although 48% of the cases could be avoided with proper management (Jo, 2020).

Research revealed 5% history of breast cancer among diabetic women and 4.2% history of prostate cancer among diabetic men. Those cancer survivors tended to be older, are less commonly treated with metformin, and had increased comorbidities compared with their cancer-free diabetic counterparts (Onitilo et al., 2013). Postmenopausal females who develop cancer of the breast also have modestly increased occurrence of diabetes among women without this cancer. The greatest risk occurs during the initial 2 years post-diagnosis, particularly among patients who had received adjuvant chemotherapy (Lipscombe et al., 2013).

The association of diabetes mellitus (DM) and risk of pancreatic cancer (PaC) has been a subject of investigation. Although it has been suggested by some that DM is not a risk factor for PaC (Gullo et al., 1994), a meta-analysis of cohort studies concluded that DM is related to an increased risk of PaC (Ben et al., 2011). The International Pancreatic Cancer Case-Control Consortium showed a 90% excess risk of PaC among people with a diagnosis of diabetes at least 2 years prior to their cancer diagnosis (Bosetti et al., 2014). Nevertheless, this risk diminishes by diabetes duration, although a 30% excess risk is seen even 20 years after diabetes diagnosis (Bosetti et al., 2014). Interestingly, prolonged oral antidiabetic drug use was linked with a reduced risk of PaC, while short-term insulin therapy raised the risk (Bosetti et al., 2014). These results indicate that DM can be both an early sign and a causative agent of PaC (Ben et al., 2011).

Interestingly, several studies have established a negative correlation between DM and prostate cancer risk. Xu et al. (2013) identified in their meta-analysis that diabetes was linked with decreased risk of prostate cancer, especially of low-grade and localized disease. Rodríguez et al. (2005) also noted a lower risk of prostate cancer in diabetic men but only some years after diabetes diagnosis. Rosenberg et al. (2002) observed a reduced risk of prostate cancer among diabetics, particularly for advanced stages, with more significant associations in white and Hispanic men. Coker et al. (2004) also observed a protective effect of diabetes on the risk of prostate cancer in older men, especially those with complications of diabetes and African-American men. These studies indicate that diabetes could have a protective effect against prostate cancer, although the association could differ depending on time since diabetes diagnosis, stage of cancer, and race.

2.3 Shared Risk Factors

The interaction between cancer and diabetes in survivors is determined by the spectrum of common risk factors, which are associated with the incidence of both disorders. These common factors tend to overlap, exerting a synergistic effect to enhance the susceptibility to diabetes in cancer survivors. Lifestyle factors feature prominently among them in determining long-term health results.

2.3.1 Lifestyle Factors

Lifestyle conditions, such as inadequate diet, lack of physical activity, obesity, and smoking, are major risk factors for both cancer and diabetes. Lifestyle changes during and after cancer treatment are common among survivors, which increase their risk of developing diabetes further. For example, chemotherapy and radiation therapy can cause fatigue, decreased mobility, and weight gain, promoting a sedentary lifestyle. In addition, depression and emotional stress, which are prevalent among survivors of cancer, may result in poor eating patterns and reduced physical activity, thereby increasing the risk further.

2.3.2 Obesity

Obesity is a key risk factor for both diabetes and most cancers, and increasing evidence corroborates the linkage between the two (Garg et al., 2013; Cifarelli & Hursting, 2015). All of the relationships between obesity, diabetes, and cancer are bridged through some interwoven pathways involving insulin resistance, hyperinsulinemia, inflammation, and sexual hormone dysregulation (Kim & Scherer, 2021). Such metabolic derangements establish a proliferation-fostering, pro-inflammatory microenvironment for cancer initiation and progression (Cifarelli & Hursting, 2015). Adipokines, pro-inflammatory cytokines, and growth factors all have essential functions in this regard, impacting signal transduction pathways and the tumor environment (Kim & Scherer, 2021). Perhaps more importantly, metabolic disturbances accompanying obesity and diabetes potentially have the effect of elevating cancer risk before diabetes becomes evident (Gallagher & Leroith, 2015a, b). Deliberate weight loss and treatments for diabetes, like metformin, could decrease cancer risk and enhance survival (Cifarelli & Hursting, 2015; Gallagher & Leroith, 2015a, b).

2.3.3 Sedentary Lifestyle

Physical inactivity has been reported to worsen obesity and metabolic disturbances, with added risks for diabetes and cancer. Sedentary behavior has become a substantial risk factor for an array of conditions, among which are diabetes and cancer. A robust amount of evidence proposes that high rates of sedentary behavior increase the risk for all-cause and cardiovascular disease mortality, together with new cases of cardiovascular disease and type 2 diabetes (Katzmarzyk et al., 2019). Physical inactivity is related to a 28–44% higher risk of colon cancer, 8–17% higher risk for breast cancer, and 28–36% for endometrial cancer (Jochem et al., 2019). Mechanisms involved between sedentary behavior and the risk of cancer are metabolic disorders, disturbances of sex hormones, and long-term inflammation (Park et al., 2020). Also, subjects with type 2 diabetes are at high risk of developing various cancers, such as colon, breast, endometrium, pancreas, and liver (Strickler et al., 2001). Hyperinsulinemia, which frequently occurs in the early phase of diabetes, may be the cause of the cancer associations of some of the risk factors, such as a sedentary lifestyle (Strickler et al., 2001).

2.3.4 Aging

Age is an important nonmodifiable risk factor for both diabetes and cancer, with advancing age being related to increased risk of these conditions (Midha et al., 2016; Vaidyanathan et al., 2016; Suh & Kim, 2019). Diabetes per se is a risk factor for numerous cancers, including pancreatic, hepatocellular, breast, and gastrointestinal cancers (Suh & Kim, 2019). The interaction between cancer, diabetes, and aging is multifaceted, with pathways including chronic inflammation, immunosenescence, hyperglycemia, and hyperinsulinemia (Suh & Kim, 2019). Obesity, a reversible risk factor, also enhances the impact of aging and further contributes to cancer risk (Midha et al., 2016). With the anticipated rise in obesity and diabetes prevalence, the understanding of these interactions is imperative for informing therapeutic strategies. Diabetic patients are advised to have regular cancer screenings since screening is lower among them despite their high risk (Midha et al., 2016; Suh & Kim, 2019). Older people have lower regenerative capacity, increased cellular senescence, and higher levels of accumulated genetic mutations that predispose them to cancer and metabolic disease.

2.3.5 Treatment-Related Factors

Cancer treatments such as chemotherapy, radiation, and endocrine therapy have the potential to induce metabolic changes. Some cancer therapies have been found to elevate diabetes risk based on newer studies. Based on a systematic review, breast cancer survivors, particularly those on tamoxifen, are at higher risk of developing type 2 diabetes (Jordt et al., 2023). The administration of corticosteroids to cancer patients was associated with a 1.29-fold increased risk of new-onset diabetes (Winn et al., 2023). Cancer treatments, including glucocorticoids, chemotherapy, and hormone therapy, may cause insulin resistance and therefore influence treatment response and disease progression (Ariaans et al., 2015). Novel cancer therapies, such as immunotherapy and targeted therapy, can also result in hyperglycemia by autoimmune β-cell destruction of pancreatic cells or through interference with insulin signaling pathways (Shariff et al., 2019).

Surprisingly, hormone therapy and chemotherapy were linked with reduced risk of new-onset diabetes in one study (Winn et al., 2023). Evidence regarding the relationship between hormone therapy for breast cancer and risk of diabetes has been inconsistent. Aromatase inhibitors or tamoxifen therapy was not found to increase the risk of diabetes in some studies in the short term (Santorelli et al., 2016). But tamoxifen use was linked to increased diabetes risk in various studies (Hamood et al., 2018; Jordt et al., 2023; Preda et al., 2024), while the effect of aromatase inhibitors is uncertain because of insufficient research (Jordt et al., 2023; Preda et al., 2024). The effect of chemotherapy on diabetes risk is also uncertain (Jordt et al., 2023; Preda et al., 2024).

3 Biological Mechanisms Linking Cancer and Diabetes

The cross talk between diabetes and cancer is controlled by multiple biological mechanisms, and insulin resistance is a key player in it. Inflammation caused by cancer, metabolic derangement, and also the action of cancer treatment all have the potential to induce derangement of insulin signaling, resulting in hyperglycemia and enhanced vulnerability to diabetes. Insulin resistance not only makes cancer survivors susceptible to diabetes but also affects cancer development because of high levels of insulin and glucose, which can potentially stimulate tumor growth. Figure 2 shows the biological mechanisms that link cancer and diabetes.

3.1 Insulin Resistance

Chemotherapy and endocrine treatment for cancer are found to cause insulin resistance, whose effect can effectively counteract the efficacy and outcome of the treatment among patients (Ariaans et al., 2015). Hyperinsulinemia brought about by insulin resistance is found to be with increased risk, incidence, and dissemination of

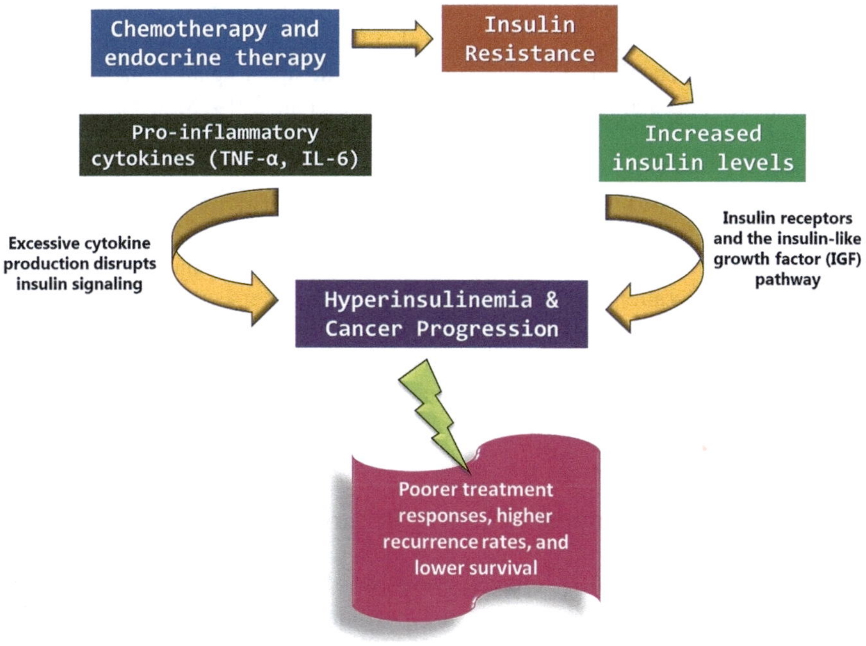

Fig. 2 Biological mechanisms linking cancer and diabetes

cancer (Szablewski, 2024). This link is especially with breast, colon, and pancreatic cancers (Cannata et al., 2010). Hyperinsulinemia can promote tumor growth by direct insulin action on insulin receptors and the insulin-like growth factor pathway (Godsland, 2009; Cannata et al., 2010). Insulin resistance and associated metabolic disturbances are also associated with poorer treatment responses, increased recurrence rates, and lower survival (Szablewski, 2024). The intricate interaction between insulin resistance, hyperinsulinemia, and cancer implies that the management of these metabolic derangements may be a future direction to optimize cancer treatment and patient prognosis (Godsland, 2009; Ariaans et al., 2015).

3.2 Inflammation

Chronic inflammation is also central to the pathogenesis of diabetes and cancer. Increased levels of pro-inflammatory cytokines, especially TNF-α and IL-6, are responsible for insulin resistance and tumor growth (Kern et al., 2018; Esser et al., 2014). IL-6, which was once thought to be mostly pro-inflammatory, has been discovered to have context-dependent actions, including anti-inflammatory properties in some contexts (Mauer et al., 2015). In obesity, inflammation in the adipose tissue results in excessive production of these cytokines, which disrupt insulin signaling and enable cancer development (Kern et al., 2018). IL-6 signaling is an important pathway through which inflammation contributes to metabolic disease and cancer (Naugler & Karin, 2008). Chronic low-grade inflammation includes immune cell infiltration within adipose tissue, liver, muscle, and pancreas, becoming pro-inflammatory in character (Esser et al., 2014). It is important to understand these inflammatory mechanisms for creating targeted therapies against obesity-related metabolic diseases and prevention of cancer (Esser et al., 2014; Mauer et al., 2015).

4 Impact of Diabetes on Cancer Survivorship

Diabetes mellitus greatly adds complexity to the path of cancer survivorship, generating a multigenerational burden for the patient. The intersection of diabetes and cancer survivorship is present in a variety of key domains, such as recurrence of cancer, decreased survival rates, and poor quality of life. Recognition of these effects is necessary to generate targeted interventions for enhancing the outcome of cancer survivors with diabetes.

4.1 Diabetes Influencing Cancer Recurrence

Hyperglycemia and insulin resistance, two of the defining characteristics of diabetes, create a pro-tumorigenic milieu that is potentially oncogenic in nature, leading to a greater risk of recurrence. A heightened blood glucose level confers a metabolic benefit to cancer cells by enhancing their growth and survival (Gallagher & LeRoith,

2015a, b). Insulin resistance also results in increased levels of insulin and insulin-like growth factor-1 (IGF-1), which are known to drive tumor progression and metastasis (Vigneri et al., 2020). These mechanisms highlight the need for glycemic control in cancer survivors with diabetes to reduce the risk of recurrence.

4.2 Diabetes and Reduced Cancer Survival Rates

Diabetic cancer survivors tend to have worse overall survival than their nondiabetic counterparts. This difference is due to the additive impact of complications from diabetes and morbidity from cancer. For example, diabetes accelerates cardiovascular disease, renal failure, and infection, all of which can weaken survival in cancer patients (Barone et al., 2008). In addition, diabetes metabolic dysregulation can lower the therapeutic effectiveness of cancer care modalities, including chemotherapy and radiation therapy, further worsening survival rates (Peairs et al., 2011).

4.3 Overburden of Diabetes in Cancer Survivors Reducing Quality of Life

The simultaneous burden of dealing with diabetes and cancer has a serious effect on the psychological and physical health of survivors. Managing diabetes involves stringent self-care measures, such as dietary limitations, frequent blood glucose monitoring, and adherence to medications, which prove daunting for people already dealing with the physical and emotional burden of cancer (Foster et al., 2019). This twofold burden tends to contribute to enhanced fatigue, depression, and anxiety, further compromising the quality of life (QoL) in this group (Pouwer et al., 2010). The resolution of these issues calls for collaborative care models that treat both conditions concurrently, with a focus on patient education, psychosocial support, and individualized treatment plans.

5 Management Strategies for Diabetes in Cancer Survivors

Optimal diabetes management in cancer survivors is best addressed through a multifaceted intervention that considers screening, lifestyle change, pharmacotherapy, and collaborative care models. These interventions could promote improved glycemic control, prevention of recurrence of cancer, and quality of life in survivors.

5.1 Screening and Early Detection

Repeated diabetes screening is vital in cancer survivors, especially high-risk populations including those with diabetes family history, obesity, and history of steroid or chemotherapy exposures. Glycated hemoglobin (HbA1c) and fasting plasma glucose examinations should be added to survivorship care plans in order to initiate early detection and timely intervention (American Diabetes Association, 2021). Identifying diabetes in its early stage enables immediate treatment, preventing its complications and providing better long-term outcomes.

5.2 Lifestyle Modifications

Lifestyle interventions play a pivotal role in managing both diabetes and cancer survivorship. These modifications not only improve glycemic control but also reduce the risk of cancer recurrence and enhance overall well-being. Balancing a diet in whole grains, vegetables, fruits, and lean protein can vastly enhance glycemic control and also inflammation, good for both the management of diabetes and cancer outcome (Rock et al., 2020). Mediterranean diets rich in plant food and healthy fat have been connected to better performance in cancer patients with diabetes (Schwingshackl et al., 2017). Regular physical activity is the cornerstone of survivorship for cancer and diabetes control. Exercise benefits cardiovascular health, reduces systemic inflammation, and increases insulin sensitivity, all of which are critical in survivors (Cormie et al., 2018). A minimum of 150 minutes of moderate-intensity exercise per week is recommended by the American Cancer Society for cancer survivors, and it can also be employed to relieve side effects of cancer therapies as well as improve quality of life (Rock et al., 2020).

5.3 Pharmacological Approaches

Careful selection of the right antidiabetic drugs is needed to prevent interference with anticancer therapy and to maximize outcomes. Certain drugs have been promising in controlling diabetes and possibly decreasing cancer-related hazards. Metformin, a first-line medication for type 2 diabetes, has been linked to decreased recurrence of cancer and enhanced survival in some types of cancer, including breast and colorectal cancer (Pollak, 2012). Its mechanisms involve decreasing insulin resistance and blocking mTOR signaling, which is involved in tumor growth. Glucagon-like peptide-1 (GLP-1) receptor agonists, including liraglutide and semaglutide, are new potential candidates for diabetes control among cancer survivors. Not only do these drugs provide better glycemic control, but they can potentially lower cancer risk because of their weight loss and anti-inflammatory properties (Drucker, 2018). Yet, more evidence is required to establish their long-term benefits among cancer survivors.

5.4 Integrated Care Models

Care models that include collaboration between oncologists, endocrinologists, primary care physicians, and other health professionals are crucial for the multidisciplinary management of diabetes in cancer survivors. Shared decision-making guarantees that treatment is individualized to the specific needs of every survivor, covering both their diabetes and cancer-specific issues (Nekhlyudov et al., 2017). Care models with integration also ensure frequent monitoring, prompt treatment changes, and better patient compliance with lifestyle and drug interventions.

6 Research Directions

The intersection of cancer survivorship and diabetes is a multifaceted and developing body of research. To enhance the prognosis of diabetes in cancer survivors, upcoming research must target elucidation of the underlying processes, exploration of personalized medicine, and longitudinal research to inform evidence-based guidelines.

6.1 Understanding Mechanisms of Cancer and Diabetes

A primary area of study is explaining the common biological pathways that connect diabetes and cancer. Hyperglycemia, insulin resistance, and chronic inflammation are major contributors to both diabetes and cancer. For example, high insulin and insulin-like growth factor-1 (IGF-1) levels in diabetes stimulate tumor growth and metastasis by activating signaling pathways such as PI3K/AKT and MAPK (Gallagher & LeRoith, 2015a, b). In addition, chronic inflammation, a characteristic feature of diabetes, generates a pro-tumorigenic microenvironment through enhanced oxidative stress and DNA damage (Giovannucci et al., 2010). Additional exploration of these processes can reveal plausible therapeutic targets that can break the diabetes-cancer connection and enhance survivorship benefits.

6.2 Personalized Medicine for Diabetes in Cancer Survivors

Personalized medicine has great potential for maximizing the care of diabetes in cancer survivors. Tailoring interventions to genetic, metabolic, and treatment-related factors can maximize the effectiveness of therapies and minimize side effects. For instance, genetic profiling can determine individuals at increased risk of developing diabetes after cancer therapy, allowing early intervention (Visscher et al., 2017). Moreover, metabolomic analysis can uncover biomarkers for predicting response to certain antidiabetic drugs, including metformin or GLP-1 receptor agonists, in the setting of cancer survivorship (Pollak, 2012). Incorporating these methods into clinical practice can result in more accurate and efficient treatment for this group.

6.3 Study of Dynamicity by Longitudinal Studies

Longitudinal research is important to decipher the dynamic relationship between cancer and diabetes over a long period of time. These types of research may give us a clue as to how diabetes impacts cancer recurrence, treatment success, and survival after a long time. For example, longitudinal research can elucidate key times of survivorship at which interventions like lifestyle changes or pharmacotherapy could be most successful (Nekhlyudov et al., 2017). In addition, such research can guide the creation of evidence-based guidelines for the care of diabetes in cancer survivors, filling gaps in present clinical practice. Large-scale cohort studies and registries are necessary to produce solid data that can inform survivorship care.

7 Conclusion

Diabetes significantly exacerbates the course of cancer survivorship, influencing recurrence rates, survival, and quality of life. The synergy between hyperglycemia, insulin resistance, and chronic inflammation creates a pro-tumorigenic environment that increases the load of cancer survivors. Diabetes care in this population is optimally managed by an integrated approach incorporating regular screening, lifestyle modification, individualized pharmacologic therapy, and coordinated care models. These interventions not only improve glycemic control but also reduce the risk of cancer recurrence and enhance quality of life. However, there are significant gaps in knowledge regarding the shared biological pathways between diabetes and cancer. Future studies will have to address these mechanisms, advance personalized medicine, and conduct longitudinal studies to guide integrated survivorship care guidelines. Through this, healthcare providers can enhance cancer survivors with diabetes, eventually contributing to their better long-term outcomes and quality of life. Further, the integration of interdisciplinary care, patient education, and innovative research will be critical in mitigating the dual burden of diabetes and cancer. As the population of cancer survivors continues to grow, prioritizing the management of diabetes in this vulnerable group is essential to ensuring they lead healthier, more fulfilling lives post-cancer treatment.

References

American Diabetes Association. (2021). Standards of medical care in diabetes—2021. *Diabetes Care, 44*(Supplement 1), S1–S232. https://doi.org/10.2337/dc21-S001

Ariaans, G., de Jong, S., Gietema, J. A., Lefrandt, J. D., de Vries, E. G. E., & Jalving, M. (2015). Cancer-drug induced insulin resistance: Innocent bystander or unusual suspect. *Cancer Treatment Reviews, 41*(4), 376–384. https://doi.org/10.1016/j.ctrv.2015.02.007

Barone, B. B., Yeh, H. C., Snyder, C. F., Peairs, K. S., Stein, K. B., Derr, R. L., Wolff, A. C., & Brancati, F. L. (2008). Long-term all-cause mortality in cancer patients with preexisting diabetes mellitus: A systematic review and meta-analysis. *JAMA, 300*(23), 2754–2764. https://doi.org/10.1001/jama.2008.824

Ben, Q., Xu, M., Ning, X., Liu, J., Hong, S., Huang, W., Zhang, H., & Li, Z. (2011). Diabetes mellitus and risk of pancreatic cancer: A meta-analysis of cohort studies. *European Journal of Cancer, 47*(13), 1928–1937. https://doi.org/10.1016/j.ejca.2011.03.003

Bizzarri, C., Bottaro, G., Pinto, R., & Cappa, M. (2019). Metabolic syndrome and diabetes mellitus in childhood cancer survivors. *Frontiers in Endocrinology, 10*, 543. https://doi.org/10.3389/fendo.2019.00543

Bosetti, C., Rosato, V., Li, D., Silverman, D. T., Petersen, G. M., Bracci, P. M., et al. (2014). Diabetes, antidiabetic medications, and pancreatic cancer risk: An analysis from the International Pancreatic Cancer Case-Control Consortium. *Annals of Oncology, 25*(10), 2065–2072. https://doi.org/10.1093/annonc/mdu276

Cannata, D., Fierz, Y., Vijayakumar, A., & Leroith, D. (2010). Type 2 diabetes and cancer: What is the connection? *The Mount Sinai Journal of Medicine, 77*(2), 197–213. https://doi.org/10.1002/msj.20161

Chueh, H., & Yoo, J. H. (2020a). Metabolic syndrome induced by anticancer treatment in childhood cancer survivors. *Journal of Pediatric Endocrinology & Metabolism, 33*(3), 309–320. https://doi.org/10.1515/jpem-2019-0530

Chueh, W. H., & Yoo, J. H. (2020b). Metabolic complications in cancer survivors: A review of the literature. *Journal of Cancer Survivorship, 14*(3), 293–303. https://doi.org/10.1007/s11764-019-00838-9

Cifarelli, V., & Hursting, S. D. (2015). Obesity, diabetes and cancer: A mechanistic perspective. *International Journal of Diabetology & Vascular Disease Research, 3*(4), 1–7. https://doi.org/10.19070/2328-353X-1500076

Coker, A. L., Sanderson, M., Zheng, W., & Fadden, M. K. (2004). Diabetes mellitus and prostate cancer risk among older men: A population-based case–control study. *British Journal of Cancer, 90*(11), 2171–2175. https://doi.org/10.1038/sj.bjc.6601749

Cormie, P., Zopf, E. M., Zhang, X., & Schmitz, K. H. (2018). The impact of exercise on cancer mortality, recurrence, and treatment-related adverse effects. *Epidemiologic Reviews, 39*(1), 71–92. https://doi.org/10.1093/epirev/mxx007

Demark-Wahnefried, W., Rogers, L. Q., Alfano, C. M., Thomson, C. A., Courneya, K. S., Meyerhardt, J. A., et al. (2017). Practical clinical interventions for diet, physical activity, and weight control in cancer survivors. *CA: a Cancer Journal for Clinicians, 67*(5), 362–377. https://doi.org/10.3322/caac.21406

DeSantis, C. E., Lin, C. C., Mariotto, A. B., Siegel, R. L., Stein, K. D., Kramer, J. L., et al. (2014). Cancer treatment and survivorship statistics, 2014. *CA: a Cancer Journal for Clinicians, 64*(4), 252–271. https://doi.org/10.3322/caac.21235

Drucker, D. J. (2018). Mechanisms of action and therapeutic application of glucagon-like peptide-1. *Cell Metabolism, 27*(4), 740–756. https://doi.org/10.1016/j.cmet.2018.03.001

Esser, N., Legrand-Poels, S., Piette, J., Scheen, A., & Paquot, N. (2014). Inflammation as a link between obesity, metabolic syndrome and type 2 diabetes. *Diabetes Research and Clinical Practice, 105*(2), 141–150. https://doi.org/10.1016/j.diabres.2014.04.006

Foster, C., Calman, L., Richardson, A., & Pimperton, H. (2019). Improving the lives of cancer survivors: A review of the evidence on supportive care needs and interventions. *Journal of Cancer Survivorship, 13*(4), 573–592. https://doi.org/10.1007/s11764-019-00784-8

Gallagher, E. J., & LeRoith, D. (2015a). Diabetes, cancer, and metformin: Connections of metabolism and cell proliferation. *Annals of the New York Academy of Sciences, 135*(1), 1–10. https://doi.org/10.1111/nyas.12907

Gallagher, E. J., & Leroith, D. (2015b). Obesity and diabetes: The increased risk of cancer and cancer-related mortality. *Physiological Reviews, 95*(3), 727–748. https://doi.org/10.1152/physrev.00030.2014

Garg, S. K., Maurer, H., Reed, K., & Selagamsetty, R. (2013). Diabetes and cancer: Two diseases with obesity as a common risk factor. *Diabetes, Obesity and Metabolism, 16*(2), 97–110. https://doi.org/10.1111/dom.12124

Giovannucci, E., Harlan, D. M., Archer, M. C., Bergenstal, R. M., Gapstur, S. M., Habel, L. A., et al. (2010). Diabetes and cancer: A consensus report. *Diabetes Care, 33*(7), 1674–1685. https://doi.org/10.2337/dc10-0666

Godsland, I. (2009). Insulin resistance and hyperinsulinaemia in the development and progression of cancer. *Clinical Science, 118*(5), 315–332. https://doi.org/10.1042/CS20090387

Gregory, J. (2018). Metabolic syndrome in cancer survivors: A growing concern. *Journal of Clinical Oncology, 36*(15), 1565–1567. https://doi.org/10.1200/JCO.2017.76.1234

Gullo, L., Pezzilli, R., & Morselli-Labate, A. M. (1994). Diabetes and the risk of pancreatic cancer. *Annals of Oncology, 5*(1), 61–63. https://doi.org/10.1093/annonc/5.1.61

Hamood, R., Hamood, H., Merhasin, I., & Keinan-Boker, L. (2018). Diabetes after hormone therapy in breast cancer survivors: A case-cohort study. *Journal of Clinical Oncology, 36*(20), 2061–2069. https://doi.org/10.1200/JCO.2017.76.3524

Hwangbo, Y. (2018). Incidence of diabetes after cancer development: A Korean national cohort study. *JAMA Oncology, 4*(8), 1099–1105. https://doi.org/10.1001/jamaoncol.2018.1684

Jo, A. (2020). New onset of type 2 diabetes as a complication after cancer diagnosis: A systematic review. *Cancer Medicine, 9*(9), 3028–3040. https://doi.org/10.1002/cam4.2932

Jochem, C., Wallmann-Sperlich, B., & Leitzmann, M. (2019). The influence of sedentary behavior on cancer risk: Epidemiologic evidence and potential molecular mechanisms. *Current Nutrition Reports, 8*(3), 167–174. https://doi.org/10.1007/s13668-019-0266-4

Jordt, N. C., Kjærgaard, K. L., Thomsen, R. W., Borgquist, S., & Cronin-Fenton, D. (2023). Breast cancer and incidence of type 2 diabetes mellitus: A systematic review and meta-analysis. *Breast Cancer Research and Treatment, 189*(3), 401–414. https://doi.org/10.1007/s10549-023-06927-8

Katzmarzyk, P. T., Powell, K. E., Jakicic, J. M., Troiano, R. P., & Piercy, K. L. (2019). Sedentary behavior and health: Update from the 2018 physical activity guidelines advisory committee. *Medicine & Science in Sports & Exercise, 51*(6), 1227–1241. https://doi.org/10.1249/MSS.0000000000001935

Kern, L., Mittenbühler, M. J., Vesting, A. J., Ostermann, A. L., Wunderlich, C. M., & Wunderlich, F. (2018). Obesity-induced TNFα and IL-6 signaling: The missing link between obesity and inflammation-driven liver and colorectal cancers. *Cancers, 10*(9), 263. https://doi.org/10.3390/cancers10090263

Kim, D.-S., & Scherer, P. (2021). Obesity, diabetes, and increased cancer progression. *Diabetes & Metabolism Journal, 45*(3), 1–14. https://doi.org/10.4093/dmj.2021.004

Lega, I. C., Pole, J. D., Austin, P. C., Lau, C., Nathan, P. C., & Baxter, N. N. (2018). Diabetes risk in childhood cancer survivors: A population-based study. *Journal of Clinical Oncology, 36*(8), 657–665. https://doi.org/10.1200/JCO.2017.76.7221

Ligibel, J. A., Alfano, C. M., Courneya, K. S., Demark-Wahnefried, W., Burger, R. A., Chlebowski, R. T., et al. (2019). American Society of Clinical Oncology position statement on obesity and cancer. *Journal of Clinical Oncology, 37*(5), 428–440. https://doi.org/10.1200/JCO.18.02477

Lipscombe, L. L., Chan, W. W., Yun, L., Austin, P. C., Anderson, G. M., & Rochon, P. A. (2013). Incidence of diabetes among postmenopausal breast cancer survivors. *Diabetologia, 56*(3), 476–483. https://doi.org/10.1007/s00125-012-2793-9

Mauer, J., Denson, J. L., & Brüning, J. (2015). Versatile functions for IL-6 in metabolism and cancer. *Trends in Immunology, 36*(2), 92–101. https://doi.org/10.1016/j.it.2014.12.008

Meacham, L. R., Sklar, C. A., Li, S., Liu, Q., Gimpel, N., Yasui, Y., et al. (2009). Diabetes mellitus in long-term survivors of childhood cancer. *Cancer, 115*(22), 4866–4874. https://doi.org/10.1200/JCO.2009.24.2267

Meacham, L. R., Sklar, C. A., Li, S., Liu, Q., Gimpel, N., Yasui, Y., et al. (2010). Diabetes mellitus in long-term survivors of childhood cancer: Increased risk associated with radiation therapy. *Journal of Clinical Oncology, 28*(7), 1260–1266. https://doi.org/10.1200/JCO.2009.24.2267

Midha, S., Chawla, S., & Garg, P. K. (2016). Modifiable and non-modifiable risk factors for pancreatic cancer: A review. *Cancer Letters, 381*(1), 269–277. https://doi.org/10.1016/j.canlet.2016.08.006

Naugler, W., & Karin, M. (2008). The wolf in sheep's clothing: The role of interleukin-6 in immunity, inflammation, and cancer. *Trends in Molecular Medicine, 14*(3), 109–119. https://doi.org/10.1016/j.molmed.2007.12.007

Nekhlyudov, L., Ganz, P. A., Arora, N. K., & Rowland, J. H. (2017). Going beyond being lost in transition: A decade of progress in cancer survivorship. *Journal of Clinical Oncology, 35*(18), 1978–1981. https://doi.org/10.1200/JCO.2016.72.1373

Oh, S., Lee, J., Hong, Y. S., & Kim, K. (2023). Increased risk of cardiovascular disease associated with diabetes among adult cancer survivors: A population-based matched cohort study. *European Journal of Preventive Cardiology, 30*(8), 670–679. https://doi.org/10.1093/eurjpc/zwad046

Onitilo, A. A., Donald, M., Stankowski, R. V., Engel, J. M., Williams, G., & Doi, S. A. (2013). Breast and prostate cancer survivors in a diabetic cohort: Results from the living with diabetes study. *Clinical Medicine & Research, 11*(4), 210–218. https://doi.org/10.3121/cmr.2013.1156

Park, J., Moon, J., Kim, H., Kong, M., & Oh, Y. (2020). Sedentary lifestyle: Overview of updated evidence of potential health risks. *Korean Journal of Family Medicine, 41*(6), 365–373. https://doi.org/10.4082/kjfm.20.0165

Peairs, K. S., Barone, B. B., Snyder, C. F., Yeh, H. C., Stein, K. B., Derr, R. L., & Brancati, F. L. (2011). Diabetes mellitus and breast cancer outcomes: A systematic review and meta-analysis. *Journal of Clinical Oncology, 29*(1), 40–46. https://doi.org/10.1200/JCO.2009.27.3011

Pollak, M. (2012). The insulin and insulin-like growth factor receptor family in neoplasia: An update. *Nature Reviews Cancer, 12*(3), 159–169. https://doi.org/10.1038/nrc3215

Pouwer, F., Nefs, G., & Nouwen, A. (2010). Diabetes and depression. *Current Diabetes Reports, 10*(6), 455–463. https://doi.org/10.1007/s11892-010-0148-9

Preda, V., Rathinam, I., Jin, L., Nguyen, A., Chen, J., & Chen, J. (2024). Systematic review of the risk of type 2 diabetes post therapy for early-stage breast cancer. *Academia Oncology, 2*(1), 34–49. https://doi.org/10.1007/s13539-024-00987-6

Rock, C. L., Thomson, C. A., Sullivan, K. R., Howe, C. L., Kushi, L. H., Caan, B. J., Neuhouser, M. L., Bandera, E. V., Wang, Y., Robien, K., Basen-Engquist, K. M., & Brown, J. C. (2020). American Cancer Society nutrition and physical activity guideline for cancer survivors. *CA: a Cancer Journal for Clinicians, 70*(4), 245–271. https://doi.org/10.3322/caac.21591

Rodriguez, C., Patel, A. V., Mondul, A. M., Jacobs, E. J., Thun, M. J., & Calle, E. E. (2005). Diabetes and risk of prostate cancer in a prospective cohort of U.S. men. *American Journal of Epidemiology, 161*(2), 147–152. https://doi.org/10.1093/aje/kwh334

Rosenberg, D. J., Neugut, A. I., Ahsan, H., & Shea, S. (2002). Diabetes mellitus and the risk of prostate cancer. *Cancer Investigation, 20*(2), 157–165. https://doi.org/10.1081/cnv-120001141

Santorelli, M. L., Hirshfield, K. M., Steinberg, M. B., Rhoads, G. G., Lin, Y., & Demissie, K. (2016). Hormonal therapy for breast cancer and diabetes incidence among postmenopausal women. *Annals of Epidemiology, 26*(5), 317–321. https://doi.org/10.1016/j.annepidem.2016.03.002

Schwingshackl, L., Schwedhelm, C., Hoffmann, G., Knüppel, S., Laure Preterre, A., Iqbal, K., Bechthold, A., De Henauw, S., Michels, N., Devleesschauwer, B., Boeing, H., & Schlesinger, S. (2017). Food groups and risk of colorectal cancer. *International Journal of Cancer, 142*(9), 1748–1758. https://doi.org/10.1002/ijc.31198

Shariff, A. I., Syed, S. A., Shelby, R. A., Force, J., Clarke, J., D'Alessio, D., & Corsino, L. (2019). Novel cancer therapies and their association with diabetes. *Journal of Molecular Endocrinology, 63*(1), R1–R15. https://doi.org/10.1530/JME-19-0054

Strickler, H. D., Wylie-Rosett, J., Rohan, T. E., Hoover, D. R., Smoller, S., Burk, R. D., & Yu, H. (2001). The relation of type 2 diabetes and cancer. *Diabetes Technology & Therapeutics, 3*(2), 263–274. https://doi.org/10.1089/152091501750281214

Suh, S., & Kim, K. (2019). Diabetes and cancer: Cancer should be screened in routine diabetes assessment. *Diabetes & Metabolism Journal, 43*(6), 733–743. https://doi.org/10.4093/dmj.2019.0187

Szablewski, L. (2024). Insulin resistance: The increased risk of cancers. *Current Oncology, 31*(1), 54–66. https://doi.org/10.3390/curroncol31020075

Vaidyanathan, V., Karunasinghe, N., Jabed, A., Pallati, R., Kao, C. H., Wang, A., Marlow, G., & Ferguson, L. (2016). Prostate cancer: Is it a battle lost to age? *Geriatrics, 1*(4), 24. https://doi.org/10.3390/geriatrics1040024

Vigneri, P., Frasca, F., Sciacca, L., Pandini, G., & Vigneri, R. (2020). Diabetes and cancer. *Endocrine-Related Cancer, 17*(4), R1–R17. https://doi.org/10.1677/ERC-09-0087

Visscher, P. M., Wray, N. R., Zhang, Q., Sklar, P., McCarthy, M. I., Brown, M. A., & Yang, J. (2017). 10 years of GWAS discovery: Biology, function, and translation. *The American Journal of Human Genetics, 101*(1), 5–22. https://doi.org/10.1016/j.ajhg.2017.06.005

Winn, M. E., Pauleck, S. P., Viskochil, R., Ulrich, C. M., Post, A. L., Richardson, S., Colman, H., Hu-Lieskovan, S., Litchman, M. L., Playdon, M. C., & Hardikar, S. (2023). Incident diabetes by obesity-related cancer status and cancer treatment type: A prospective study using electronic medical records data. *Cancer Epidemiology, Biomarkers & Prevention, 32*(4), 455–465. https://doi.org/10.1158/1055-9965.EPI-22-0853

Xiao, Y., Wang, H., Tang, Y., Yan, J., Cao, L., Chen, Z., Shao, Z., Mei, Z., & Jiang, Z. (2021). Increased risk of diabetes in cancer survivors: A pooled analysis of 13 population-based cohort studies. *ESMO Open, 6*, 100218. https://doi.org/10.1016/j.esmoop.2021.100218

Xu, H., Jiang, H., Ding, G., Zhang, H., Zhang, L., Mao, S., & Ding, Q. (2013). Diabetes mellitus and prostate cancer risk of different grade or stage: A systematic review and meta-analysis. *Diabetes Research and Clinical Practice, 99*(3), 241–249. https://doi.org/10.1016/j.diabres.2012.12.003

Strategies for Reducing the Risk of Diabetes and Cancer

Arumugam Kamaladevi, Mamali Das, Chandramohan Kiruthiga, and K. Langeswaran

Abstract

The increased global burden of diabetes mellitus and cancer has necessitated a paradigm shift toward preventive, integrative, and evidence-driven strategies targeting their shared etiological determinants. This chapter presents an in-depth analysis of scientifically validated interventions aimed at mitigating the dual risk of these chronic diseases through lifestyle modification, metabolic regulation, and behavioral restructuring. The chapter also emphasizes the mechanistic role of dietary composition, energy balance, and adiposity control in interrupting the mechanisms linking metabolic dysfunction with carcinogenesis. The chapter elucidates how diets enriched with whole grains, fruits, vegetables, polyphenols, omega-3 fatty acids, and antioxidants counteract hyperinsulinemia, oxidative stress, and chronic inflammation, which are the key molecular drivers of both diabetes and tumor development. In contrast, excess consumption of saturated fats, processed foods, and alcohol, alongside physical inactivity, contributes to insulin resistance, adipose tissue dysfunction, and systemic inflammatory signaling that fosters a pro-tumorigenic environment. Furthermore, the chapter examines the impact of obesity as a metabolic and hormonal disruptor that alters cytokine profiles, induces DNA damage through reactive oxygen species, and modulates growth factor pathways that are implicated in oncogenesis. The chapter also focuses on the beneficial role of Mediterranean diet and aerobic and resistance-based physical activity as an important strategy for disease prevention. The integration of these interventions into personalized healthcare models, public health policies, and clinical practice is an important factor for curbing the interlinked epidemics of diabetes and cancer. Toward the end, the chapter presents a translational perspective that unites molecular understanding with public

A. Kamaladevi · M. Das · C. Kiruthiga · K. Langeswaran (✉)
Department of Biomedical Science, Science Campus, Alagappa University, Karaikudi, Tamil Nadu, India

R. Noor (ed.), *Diabetes and Cancer: Association, Mechanism, and Therapeutic Implications*, https://doi.org/10.1007/978-981-95-5651-9_5

health implementation, advancing a healthcare model that prioritizes prevention over treatment in managing intertwined metabolic and neoplastic disorders.

Keywords

Metabolic syndrome · Lifestyle interventions · Insulin resistance · Oxidative stress · Chronic inflammation · Obesity · Glycemic control · Physical activity · Metformin · Preventive medicine

1 Introduction

Globally, public health systems have been seriously threatened by noncommunicable diseases like cancer and diabetes (WHO, https://www.who.int/news-room/fact-sheets/detail/noncommunicable-diseases, 2024) Comprehensive strategies that emphasize modifiable risk factors and encourage early detection and intervention are required in light of the startlingly high prevalence of diabetes and cancer. To mitigate the risk factors, comprehensive and targetd intern=ventions are required. According to Shahid et al. (2021), current treatment strategies have limited potential in limiting the incidence of diabetes and cancer. Lifestyle modifications hold tremendous potential for improving public health outcomes by decreasing major metabolic risk factors, including obesity, gaining weight, blood glucose, blood pressure, and blood lipids (Santos, 2022), to manage the diseases and its comorbidity.

2 Reducing the Risk of Cancer

Cancer, a major cause of death, has been defined by the unchecked proliferation and spread of aberrant cells. Targeted interventions have the potential to prevent cancer because a considerable percentage of cases are linked to modifiable risk factors (Santos, 2022).

2.1 Lifestyle Modifications to Prevent Cancer

According to the World Health Organization (WHO), health is more than just the absence of sickness; it also includes mental, social, and physical well-being. Control, organization, and selection of all behaviors that may affect a person's health are required to reach this state. This kind of health growth and maintenance is known as a healthy lifestyle (Fig. 1), which encompasses both disease prevention and the adoption of lifelong well-being-promoting habits (Bostan & Beşer, 2017). Among the fundamental components of a healthy lifestyle include behaviors like eating in moderation and in a way that is acceptable, managing stress, engaging in regular and moderate physical activity, and quitting smoking (Çetinkaya & Sert, 2021).

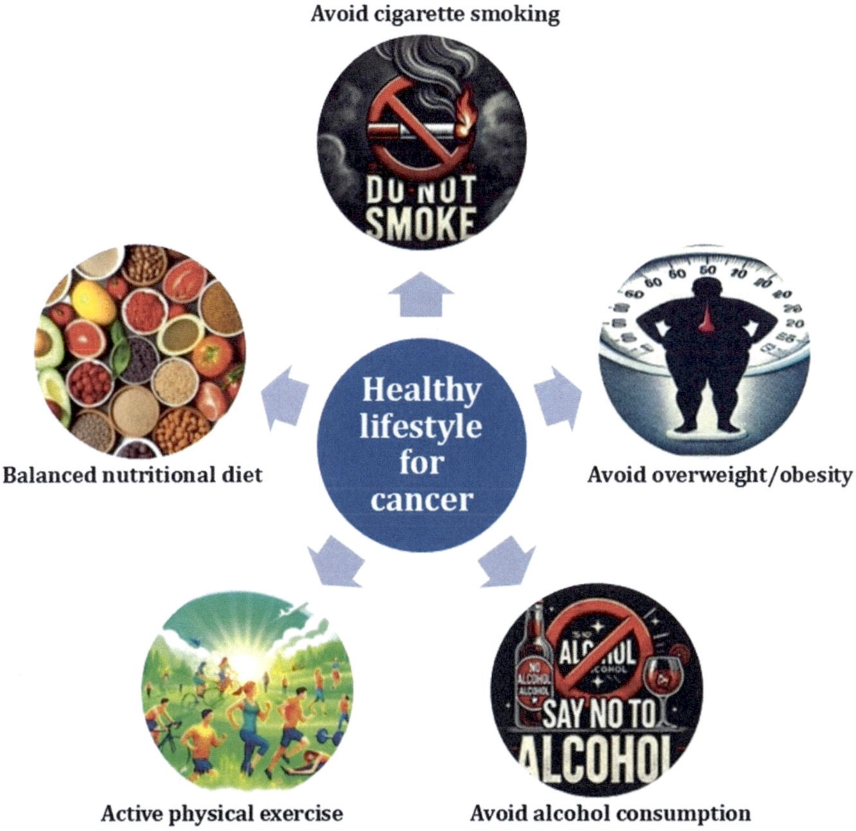

Fig. 1 Healthy lifestyle to prevent cancer

2.1.1 Dietary Strategies

The dietary approach has been a widely recognized key component that is linked to cancer genesis and prevention. Extensive epidemiology studies both in vivo and in vitro significantly evidenced the link between dietary choices and risk of cancer (Khan et al., 2018; Ruiz & Hernández, 2014). For instance, it has been demonstrated that a nutritional diet rich in fiber, vegetables, and fruits with micronutrients helps protect cancer. Conversely, consuming excessive fat and alcohol may increase the chance of cancer genesis (Hinduja et al., 2023). It has been found that consuming healthy diet reduces and prevents the development of cancer by 30–50% (Vineis & Wild, 2014). On the other hand, mounting evidences also demonstrated the indirect association of cancer risk with ingesting vegetables, fruits, whole grains, n-3 fatty acids, etc. (Morze et al., 2021). However, Glade (1999) deciphered the association of excessive intake of animal-derived saturated fat, alcohol, and obesity to cancer risk. In addition, Greenwald et al. (2001) have also substantiated the prominence of dietary fiber, vegetables, fruits, and physical activities in preventing cancer risks. Another cohort study stated that modifiable risk factors such as obesity, consumption of red meat, alcohol intake, cigarette smoking, and inadequate folic acid during early adulthood have a higher risk of colon cancer than a healthier lifestyle (Platz et al., 2000).

Remarkably, polyphenolic substances are renowned for their ability to prevent cancer. Numerous studies have demonstrated the protective effects of diets high in fiber, fruits, vegetables, polyphenolic compounds, carotenoids, vitamin B12, milk, and dairy products against malignancies of the stomach, breast, colon, prostate, and esophagus (Solans et al., 2018; Fliss-Isakov et al., 2018; Farràs et al., 2021). Dietary foods' anticancer properties are mostly ascribed to their anti-inflammatory and antioxidant properties, as well as the potential of their bioactive components to promote apoptosis and prevent inflammation, angiogenesis, cancer cell proliferation, and invasiveness (Lăcătuşu et al., 2019; Muffone et al., 2023). The Mediterranean diet generally rich in bioactive components is regarded as one of the healthiest diets (Lăcătuşu et al., 2019, Muffone et al., 2023). Consequently, consistent Mediterranean diet intake has significantly reduced the incidence and mortality of colon, breast, prostate, stomach, head, and liver diseases (Schwingshackl et al., 2017; Kuan et al., 2019; Hashemian et al., 2019). Table 1 presents the list of food or bioactive elements that prevent different types of cancer.

2.1.2 Obesity and Overweight

In addition to being the leading cause of cancer (Siegel et al., 2023), obesity and a high body mass index (BMI) increase risk for both men and women (Sung et al., 2019). According to study conducted among adults, obesity accounts for 10% of cancer incidence in women as well as 5% in men (Islami et al., 2019; Ugai et al., 2022). The mechanisms by which body weight and obesity increase the chance of acquiring different types of cancer have been elucidated by numerous studies. It has been demonstrated that carrying too much weight causes abnormalities in adipose tissue, which stimulate the release of cytokines like TNF and interleukine-6. Additionally, an imbalance in adipose tissue encourages chronic inflammation,

Table 1 The list of food or bioactive elements that prevent different types of cancer

Compound	Types of cancer	References
Polyphenol, carotenoids, vitamin B12, folic acid, selenium, fiber-rich food, omega-3 fatty acid-rich nuts and oily fish	Colorectal, breast, stomach, prostate, esophageal	Solans et al. (2018), Fliss-Isakov et al. (2018), Farràs et al. (2021)
Food that lacks saturated and unsaturated fat, green tea, (−)-epigallocatechin-3-gallate	Breast cancer	Dandamudi et al. (2018), Choi and Hua (2021), Zhang et al. (2020), Ratnani and Malik (2022)
Vitamins; polyphenols; folic acid; lycopene; β-carotenoid in pumpkin, carrot, and tomatoes; green tea; catechins; and epicatechins	Colorectal cancer	Marino et al. (2023), Hori et al. (2023), Kumar et al. (2023)
n-3 eicosapentaenoic acid, Mediterranean diet, potatoes, cereals, beans, seeds, nuts, oleic acid, and omega-3 fatty acid	Prostate cancer	Pelser et al. (2013), Capurso and Vendemiale (2017), Bilodeau et al. (2021)

which raises the risk of cancer (Célind et al., 2022). A cellular environment with elevated oxidative stress and reactive oxygen species which damages DNA is another significant mechanism associated with obesity. Due to the insufficient intake of a nutritious diet high in antioxidants, the excess of ROS also plays a role in carcinogenesis (Włodarczyk & Nowicka, 2019; Hayes et al., 2020; Maiuolo et al., 2021). Uncontrolled hormone synthesis, including growth hormones, leptin, estrogens, and androgens in women, is another mechanism behind the emergence of different types of cancer (Spyrou et al., 2018; Almendros et al., 2020). Additionally, studies have demonstrated that losing weight protects against cancer and improves the quality of existing treatments (Harris et al., 2022). According to another research, obesity raises the chance of recurrence and death for individuals who have already recovered from cancer in addition to being associated with the risk of contracting the disease (Aune et al., 2016; Petrelli et al., 2021). For this reason, dietary education must be implemented to stop the onset of different kinds of cancer.

Overweight and obesity have been linked to breast cancer in numerous analyses (Kerlikowske et al., 2017). Adipose tissue increases the risk of tumor growth because it serves as a major source of estrogen, particularly in menopausal women (Chen et al., 2016; Miller et al., 2018). A meta-analysis revealed that postmenopausal women with higher body weight displayed 82% greater risk of developing ER-positive breast cancer compared to women with lower body weight (van den Brandt et al., 2021). Furthermore, weight gain in young women significantly involved 17% of ER+/PR+ postmenopausal breast cancer (Rosner et al., 2017). According to the statistics, women who weigh too little over a 10–20-year period have a decreased chance of getting breast cancer (Sangrajrang et al., 2013; Youn & Han, 2020). Women with a higher body mass index of 30 kg/m^2 were observed to have lower overall survival and disease-free survival than women with a normal weight (Scholz et al., 2015).

Astonishingly, developing colorectal cancer is associated with overweight (BMI $\geq$ 25–30 kg/m^2) or obesity (BMI $\geq$ 30 kg/m^2). Recent studies deciphered that developing colorectal cancer is about 18% higher for overweight people and 32% higher for obese people than for normal-weight people (Zhang et al., 2021; Lei et al., 2021). According to an analysis, increased BMI of 8 kg/m^2 raises the chance of acquiring cancer to 10% (Johnson et al., 2013), and 5 kg rise in weight increases the chance by 3% (Rawla et al., 2019).

Additionally, a 4% higher risk of colorectal cancer is associated with 2 cm increase in waist circumference (Bhaskaran et al., 2018; Chaplin et al., 2022). However, some research indicates that weight loss may mitigate the risk of colorectal cancer progression (Tzenios, 2023). The interlink of obesity and prostate cancer is still up for dispute. Obesity and the incidence of prostate cancer have been reported to be directly correlated in certain studies but not in others (Mandic et al., 2023).

2.1.3 Physical Activity

It has been demonstrated that exercise can prevent cancer. Specifically, a wealth of evidence shows that physical activity lowers the incidence of lung, ovarian, kidney, and pancreatic cancers and the risk of several cancers, including colorectal, endometrial, esophageal, stomach, bladder, and breast cancers (Clemente-Suárez et al., 2023b). Accordingly, exercise alleviates the risk of cancer by 10–25% (McTiernan et al., 2019). Regular physical activity and a healthy lifestyle are associated with higher existence for cancer survivors (Van Blarigan et al., 2018; Friedenreich et al., 2020). The potential of exercise to affect inflammation and the immune system seems to be the most significant mechanism behind the benefits of physical activity. On the other hand, inactive lifestyle weakens the immune system, causes inflammation, and raises the development of cancer. Also, lesser exercise pays the way for the accumulation of fat under adipose tissue and triggers inflammatory factors that lead to chronic inflammation, which in turn fuels the formation of tumors (Wang & Zhou, 2021; Clemente-Suárez et al., 2023a, b).

Research has shown that engaging in physical activity can help prevent breast cancer (Chen et al., 2019; Boraka et al., 2022). According to a clinical study conducted on postmenopausal women aged 50–79, engaging in active physical activity showed decreased risk of cancer in breast (McTiernan et al., 2004). Furthermore, breast cancer women who regularly exercised throughout the week had a lower risk of dying from the disease (Holick et al., 2008; Kim et al., 2015). Likely, active exercise probably lowers the colorectal cancer by 12% for women and 19% for men (Xie et al., 2021).

2.1.4 Alcohol Consumption

Globally, alcohol consumption poses a major public health issue. Its characteristic chemicals are a highly hazardous chemical and a group I carcinogen that causes a variety of cancers, such as breast, colorectal, liver, and esophageal cancers (Bostan et al., 2017). It accounts for an annual cause of approximately 4% or 740,000 malignancy cases (Rumgay et al., 2021). Breast, liver, and esophageal cancers are the primary cancers in alcohol consumers. For these reasons, improving alcohol consumption prevention is one of the global goals. The discussion about alcohol consumption is paradoxical. Some studies have found that even moderate alcohol consumption may increase the incidence of malignancies of the mouth, esophagus, liver, breast, and colon (McNabb et al., 2020; Klein et al., 2020). Conversely, it has been demonstrated that moderate alcohol consumption reduces the incidence of cancer (Bagnardi et al., 2015). In lieu of this, another research found that patients who consume less alcohol showed lower risk of cancer than normal individuals (Li et al., 2018). These results supported the idea that a Mediterranean diet that includes moderate amounts of red wine at meals can significantly reduce the risk of cancer (Ventriglio et al., 2020; Jani et al., 2021).

2.1.5 Smoking

Smoking cigarettes is one of the principal risk factors for developing cancer and the leading causes of cancer death. Numerous studies have established the link between smoking cigarettes and lung cancer (Adams et al., 2023; Leiter et al., 2023). Smoking has been significantly related to cancers of the head and neck, bladder, cervix, stomach, colon, esophagus, pancreas, kidney, and liver according to substantial evidence (Adams et al., 2023, Leiter et al., 2023). Additionally, other research has demonstrated that chronic smokers are more likely to acquire cancer (Smith et al., 2019; Krutz et al., 2022). Additionally, it has been demonstrated that individuals who continue cigarette after receiving a cancer diagnosis are at an increased risk of dying from respiratory and cardiovascular issues associated with smoking, as well as an increased incidence of tumor recurrence, intervention complications, and the development of new primary tumors (Gritz et al., 2020; Sheikh et al., 2021).

3 Reducing the Risk of Diabetes

Diabetes mellitus (DM) poses serious threats on individuals, healthcare systems, economy, and societies, globally. It has been accounted that about 7% of people have prediabetes and 8% have diabetes. Among diabetic patients, 95% were observed to have DM. Numerous studies have shown that lifestyle intervention programs that promote a balanced diet, regular exercise, and modest weight loss can either prevent the diabetes in high-risk patients, including those with impaired glucose tolerance (Balk et al., 2015; Gong et al., 2015). Drug-based therapies for diabetes are only partially effective in long-term management. In order achieve optimal disease management, patients need to implement a significant lifestyle change in addition to medication interventions. These usually involve dietary adjustments, physical exercise, stress management or related issues, and better sleep habits.

3.1 Dietary Interventions

High consumption of sweets, fried foods, and red meat is strongly linked with insulin resistance and development of DM (Clemente-Suárez et al., 2023a, b). Conversely, eating vegetables that are strong in antioxidants, fiber, and other nutrients is associated with a decreased risk of developing diabetes (Villegas et al., 2008; Abdali et al., 2015). Obese patients with diabetes have different average energy intakes. It is generally advised that nonobese diabetic patients consume 1500–2500 calories daily on average, while obese patients should consume an average of 800–1500 calories daily. Patients with DM should limit their consumption of processed sugars. For these people, sugar can be effectively replaced with nonnutritive sweeteners such as aspartame, saccharine, etc. Additionally, it is recommended to restrict consumption of foods that are high in cholesterol and saturated fats and replace them with foods rich in polyunsaturated fats. Furthermore, limiting potential postprandial spikes in blood glucose levels can be achieved by altering eating habits, such as splitting meals into smaller portions throughout the day as opposed to consuming one or two large meals (Asif, 2014). A decreased incidence of diabetes is substantially linked to strict adherence to a regulated diet and enough physical activity. Diabetic patients' ability to handle glucose is significantly improved when they adopt a Paleolithic diet, which is high in lean meat, fish, fruits, and vegetables (Kirwan et al., 2017).

Indians suggested that diet played a vital role in the aetiology of type 2 diabetes after observing that the condition was more common among wealthy individuals who consumed large amount of sugar, flour, and oil (Lin & Li, 2021). According to them, there is a robust correlation between excessive carbohydrate and fat intake and DM. Accordingly, food shortages and famines during World Wars I and II caused declines in diabetes mortality rates in Germany, European countries, and Berlin. However, in other countries that did not experience a food shortage during the same period, such as Japan and North American countries, the diabetes mortality rate remained unchanged (Sami et al., 2017). Numerous studies have also shown a link between the development of DM and a high sugar intake (Khatib, 2004). A study by Ludwig et al. (2001) with 500 students from a variety of ethnic backgrounds discovered that the frequency of obesity rose with each additional serving of carbonated drinks. Recent research has indicated a connection between soft drink use and diabetes and obesity. The hazardous effect of soft drinks is attributed to the significant amounts of high-fructose corn syrup, which boosts blood glucose and body mass index to dangerously high levels (Nseir et al., 2010). Additionally, glycated compounds found in diet soft drinks significantly increase insulin resistance that leads to DM. A high consumption of fried meals, sweets, and red meat raises the risk of insulin resistance and DM. On the other hand, there was a negative relationship found between vegetable consumption and DM. Because fruits and vegetables are high in nutrients, fiber, and antioxidants that act as a barrier against diseases, thus, consuming them may help prevent the development of DM. According to a recent study, Japanese women who eat more white rice had a greater incidence of DM (Nanri et al., 2010). This calls for a significant change in the way of life of the general populace as well as a better awareness of healthy eating practices worldwide.

3.2 Physical Activity and Exercise

Exercise and physical activity was positively correlated with hyperglycemia levels in DM patients. It has been discovered that regular, moderate physical activities like walking, gardening, and doing routine household are a useful strategy for managing the long-term effects of diabetes. The best physical activity for people with DM is walking because it helps patients who are already physically weak achieve significant glucose control with little physical strain. Furthermore, alterations in sedentary behavior are a highly justified lifestyle adjustment for individuals with DM. Sedentary lifestyles result in significantly lower energy expenditure. Likely, uncontrolled glucose levels in DM patients are also linked to prolonged periods of inactivity. Regular aerobic exercise has also been shown to lower HbA1c levels in diabetic patients (Snowling & Hopkins, 2006). In addition, aerobic workouts improve several outcomes in patients through multifaceted mechanism such as higher insulin sensitivity, improved lung functions, and increased mitochondrial densities (Garber et al., 2011). Therefore, reducing inactive time is essential for diabetics, and this can be accomplished by increased physical activity.

3.3 Stress

In DM patients, elevated stress levels are linked to poor glycemic control and compliance with medications. Moderate to high levels of stress were found to be responsible for a multifold increase in the risk of diabetes in a longitudinal investigation (Vasanth et al., 2017). Furthermore, psychological stress, weakened mental health, and prolonged exposure to stressors are strongly linked to an increased risk of developing diabetes. It is believed that the main cause of this elevated risk of DM in these people is allostatic load, or physical deterioration brought on by ongoing psychological stress (Kelly & Ismail, 2015). Furthermore, persistent stress is linked to a decline in the clinical results of individuals with diabetes mellitus. Low-grade inflammation and dysregulated glucose metabolism and neuroendocrine function are linked to chronic stress. Psychological stress has a significant impact on most of the parameters linked to DM, such as the release of glucose (and lipids) into the bloodstream, the development of inflammatory cytokines, and high blood pressure. In one investigation, significant increases in blood glucose levels were noted in patients with DM, who experienced acute stress during the postprandial period (Hackett & Steptoe, 2017). The occurrence of DM appears to be efficiently prevented or controlled by therapeutic measures, such as stress management therapies.

3.4 Sleep Behavior

Despite the fact that exercise and a healthy diet lead to significant gains in the management of DM, they cannot be considered the only factors contributing to the rise in diabetes cases. Another lifestyle choice that can be changed that has been shown to affect energy levels and metabolic health is sleep. In order to control diabetes, sleep patterns must be optimized (Arora & Taheri, 2015). According to a population-based study, insomnia or short sleep duration (less than 5 h) may be linked to a higher risk of DM. Similar studies found that DM patients with inadequate sleep had higher HbA1c levels (>7%) and insulin resistance (Vgontzas et al., 2009). The incidence, progression, and treatment of diabetes are also significantly impacted by disrupted circadian rhythms and sleep-wake patterns (Arora & Taheri, 2015). Due to frequent sleep deprivation and irregular circadian rhythms, shift workers are more likely to develop metabolic problems (De Bacquer et al., 2009). Furthermore, a significant risk of DM is linked to a developed tendency to nap as a result of inadequate or poor nocturnal sleep. In a previous study, the insulin response to a standardized meal was significantly reduced as a result of systematically manipulating sleep and circadian cycles; this effect may be regained with the restoration of sleeping patterns. Likely, insufficient sleep has been linked to changes in the hormones leptin and ghrelin, which control hunger. These changes enhance the appetite for foods high in carbohydrates and thus increase caloric intake (Taheri et al., 2004). Additionally, sleep deprivation causes oxidative stress and leads to the release of orexin or hypocretin, a neuropeptide that controls appetite and sleep, stimulates the sympathetic nervous system, increases cortisol release, and concurrently decreases growth hormone secretion, all of which contribute to significant hyperglycemia, which ultimately leads to DM (Arora & Taheri, 2015).

References

Abdali, D., Samson, S. E., & Grover, A. K. (2015). How effective are antioxidant supplements in obesity and diabetes? *Medical Principles and Practice, 24*(3), 201–215.

Adams, S. J., Stone, E., Baldwin, D. R., Vliegenthart, R., Lee, P., & Fintelmann, F. J. (2023). Lung cancer screening. *The Lancet, 401*(10374), 390–408.

Almendros, I., Martinez-Garcia, M. A., Farré, R., & Gozal, D. (2020). Obesity, sleep apnea, and cancer. *International Journal of Obesity, 44*(8), 1653–1667.

Arora, T., & Taheri, S. (2015). Sleep optimization and diabetes control: A review of the literature. *Diabetes Therapy, 6*, 425–468.

Asif, M. (2014). The prevention and control the type-2 diabetes by changing lifestyle and dietary pattern. *Journal of Education and Health Promotion, 3*(1), 1.

Aune, D., Sen, A., Prasad, M., Norat, T., Janszky, I., Tonstad, S., et al. (2016). BMI and all cause mortality: Systematic review and non-linear dose-response meta-analysis of 230 cohort studies with 3.74 million deaths among 30.3 million participants. *BMJ (Clinical research ed.), 353*.

Bagnardi, V., Rota, M., Botteri, E., Tramacere, I., Islami, F., Fedirko, V., et al. (2015). Alcohol consumption and site-specific cancer risk: A comprehensive dose–response meta-analysis. *British Journal of Cancer, 112*(3), 580–593.

Balk, E. M., Earley, A., Raman, G., Avendano, E. A., Pittas, A. G., & Remington, P. L. (2015). Combined diet and physical activity promotion programs to prevent type 2 diabetes among persons at increased risk: A systematic review for the Community Preventive Services Task Force. *Annals of Internal Medicine, 163*(6), 437–451.

Bhaskaran, K., dos-Santos-Silva, I., Leon, D. A., Douglas, I. J., & Smeeth, L. (2018). Association of BMI with overall and cause-specific mortality: A population-based cohort study of 3·6 million adults in the UK. *The Lancet Diabetes & Endocrinology, 6*(12), 944–953.

Bilodeau, J. F., Gevariya, N., Larose, J., Robitaille, K., Roy, J., Oger, C., et al. (2021). Long chain omega-3 fatty acids and their oxidized metabolites are associated with reduced prostate tumor growth. *Prostaglandins, Leukotrienes and Essential Fatty Acids, 164*, 102215.

Boraka, Ö., Klintman, M., & Rosendahl, A. H. (2022). Physical activity and long-term risk of breast cancer, associations with time in life and body composition in the prospective Malmö diet and cancer study. *Cancers, 14*(8), 1960.

Bostan, N., & Beşer, A. (2017). Factors affecting the healthy lifestyle behaviors of nurses. *Journal of Education and Research in Nursing, 14*(1), 38–44.

Capurso, C., & Vendemiale, G. (2017). The Mediterranean diet reduces the risk and mortality of the prostate cancer: A narrative review. *Frontiers in Nutrition, 4*, 38.

Célind, J., Bygdell, M., Martikainen, J., Ohlsson, C., & Kindblom, J. M. (2022). Childhood overweight and risk of obesity-related adult cancer in men. *Cancer Communications, 42*(6), 576.

Çetinkaya, S., & Sert, H. (2021). Healthy lifestyle behaviors of university students and related factors. *Acta Paulista de Enfermagem, 34*, eAPE02942.

Chaplin, A., Rodriguez, R. M., Segura-Sampedro, J. J., Ochogavía-Seguí, A., Romaguera, D., & Barceló-Coblijn, G. (2022). Insights behind the relationship between colorectal cancer and obesity: Is visceral adipose tissue the missing link? *International Journal of Molecular Sciences, 23*(21), 13128.

Chen, M. J., Wu, W. Y., Yen, A. M., Fann, J. C., Chen, S. L., Chiu, S. Y., et al. (2016). Body mass index and breast cancer: Analysis of a nation-wide population-based prospective cohort study on 1 393 985 Taiwanese women. *International Journal of Obesity, 40*(3), 524–530.

Chen, X., Wang, Q., Zhang, Y., Xie, Q., & Tan, X. (2019). Physical activity and risk of breast cancer: A meta-analysis of 38 cohort studies in 45 study reports. *Value in Health, 22*(1), 104–128.

Choi, J. W., & Hua, T. N. (2021). Impact of lifestyle behaviors on cancer risk and prevention. *Journal of Lifestyle Medicine, 11*(1), 1.

Clemente-Suárez, V. J., Beltrán-Velasco, A. I., Redondo-Flórez, L., Martín-Rodríguez, A., & Tornero-Aguilera, J. F. (2023a). Global impacts of western diet and its effects on metabolism and health: A narrative review. *Nutrients, 15*(12), 2749.

Clemente-Suárez, V. J., Martín-Rodríguez, A., Redondo-Flórez, L., Ruisoto, P., Navarro-Jiménez, E., Ramos-Campo, D. J., & Tornero-Aguilera, J. F. (2023b). Metabolic health, mitochondrial fitness, physical activity, and cancer. *Cancers, 15*(3), 814.

Dandamudi, A., Tommie, J., Nommsen-Rivers, L., & Couch, S. (2018). Dietary patterns and breast cancer risk: A systematic review. *Anticancer Research, 38*(6), 3209–3222.

De Bacquer, D., Van Risseghem, M., Clays, E., Kittel, F., De Backer, G., & Braeckman, L. (2009). Rotating shift work and the metabolic syndrome: A prospective study. *International Journal of Epidemiology, 38*(3), 848–854.

Farràs, M., Almanza-Aguilera, E., Hernáez, Á., Agustí, N., Julve, J., Fitó, M., & Castañer, O. (2021, August). Beneficial effects of olive oil and Mediterranean diet on cancer physio-pathology and incidence. In *Seminars in Cancer Biology* (Vol. 73, pp. 178–195). Academic Press.

Fliss-Isakov, N., Kariv, R., Webb, M., Ivancovsky, D., Margalit, D., & Zelber-Sagi, S. (2018). Mediterranean dietary components are inversely associated with advanced colorectal polyps: A case-control study. *World Journal of Gastroenterology, 24*(24), 2617.

Friedenreich, C. M., Stone, C. R., Cheung, W. Y., & Hayes, S. C. (2020). Physical activity and mortality in cancer survivors: A systematic review and meta-analysis. *JNCI Cancer Spectrum, 4*(1), pkz080.

Garber, C. E., Blissmer, B., Deschenes, M. R., Franklin, B. A., Lamonte, M. J., Lee, I. M., et al. (2011). Quantity and quality of exercise for developing and maintaining cardiorespiratory, musculoskeletal, and neuromotor fitness in apparently healthy adults: Guidance for prescribing exercise. *Medicine and Science in Sports and Exercise, 43*(7), 1334–1359.

Glade, M. J. (1999). Food, nutrition, and the prevention of cancer: A global perspective. American institute for cancer research/world cancer research fund, American institute for cancer research, 1997. *Nutrition, 15*, 523–526.

Gong, Q. H., Kang, J. F., Ying, Y. Y., Li, H., Zhang, X. H., Wu, Y. H., & Xu, G. Z. (2015). Lifestyle interventions for adults with impaired glucose tolerance: A systematic review and meta-analysis of the effects on glycemic control. *Internal Medicine, 54*(3), 303–310.

Greenwald, P., Clifford, C. K., & Milner, J. A. (2001). Diet and cancer prevention. *European Journal of Cancer, 37*(8), 948–965.

Gritz, E. R., Talluri, R., Domgue, J. F., Tami-Maury, I., & Shete, S. (2020). Smoking behaviors in survivors of smoking-related and non–smoking-related cancers. *JAMA Network Open, 3*(7), e209072.

Hackett, R. A., & Steptoe, A. (2017). Type 2 diabetes mellitus and psychological stress—A modifiable risk factor. *Nature Reviews Endocrinology, 13*(9), 547–560.

Harris, B. H., Macaulay, V. M., Harris, D. A., Klenerman, P., Karpe, F., Lord, S. R., et al. (2022). Obesity: A perfect storm for carcinogenesis. *Cancer and Metastasis Reviews, 41*(3), 491–515.

Hashemian, M., Farvid, M. S., Poustchi, H., Murphy, G., Etemadi, A., Hekmatdoost, A., et al. (2019). The application of six dietary scores to a Middle Eastern population: A comparative analysis of mortality in a prospective study. *European Journal of Epidemiology, 34*, 371–382.

Hayes, J. D., Dinkova-Kostova, A. T., & Tew, K. D. (2020). Oxidative stress in cancer. *Cancer Cell, 38*(2), 167–197.

Hinduja, D. B., Dhanu, A., Swamy, G., Murugesan, K., Elango, B., Murali, U., et al. (2023). Diet and nutrition strategies for cancer prevention: A comprehensive review. *Research in Biotechnology, 2023*(14), 12–18.

Holick, C. N., Newcomb, P. A., Trentham-Dietz, A., Titus-Ernstoff, L., Bersch, A. J., Stampfer, M. J., et al. (2008). Physical activity and survival after diagnosis of invasive breast cancer. *Cancer Epidemiology Biomarkers & Prevention, 17*(2), 379–386.

Hori, M., Sawada, N., Kito, K., Yamaji, T., Iwasaki, M., Inoue, M., & Tsugane, S. (2023). Vegetable and fruit intake and colorectal cancer risk by smoking status in adults: The Japan public health center-based prospective study. *European Journal of Clinical Nutrition, 77*(2), 255–263.

https://www.who.int/news-room/fact-sheets/detail/noncommunicable-diseases (2024).

Islami, F., Sauer, A. G., Gapstur, S. M., & Jemal, A. (2019). Proportion of cancer cases attributable to excess body weight by US state, 2011-2015. *JAMA Oncology, 5*(3), 384–392.

Jani, B. D., McQueenie, R., Nicholl, B. I., Field, R., Hanlon, P., Gallacher, K. I., et al. (2021). Association between patterns of alcohol consumption (beverage type, frequency and consumption with food) and risk of adverse health outcomes: A prospective cohort study. *BMC Medicine, 19*, 1–14.

Johnson, C. M., Wei, C., Ensor, J. E., Smolenski, D. J., Amos, C. I., Levin, B., & Berry, D. A. (2013). Meta-analyses of colorectal cancer risk factors. *Cancer Causes & Control, 24*, 1207–1222.

Kelly, S. J., & Ismail, M. (2015). Stress and type 2 diabetes: A review of how stress contributes to the development of type 2 diabetes. *Annual Review of Public Health, 36*(1), 441–462.

Kerlikowske, K., Gard, C. C., Tice, J. A., Ziv, E., Cummings, S. R., Miglioretti, D. L., & Breast Cancer Surveillance Consortium. (2017). Risk factors that increase risk of estrogen receptor–positive and–negative breast cancer. *Journal of the National Cancer Institute, 109*(5), djw276.

Khan, H., Khan, M. S., & Ahmad, S. (2018). The in vivo and in vitro approaches for establishing a link between advanced glycation end products and lung cancer. *Journal of Cellular Biochemistry, 119*(11), 9099–9109.

Khatib, O. (2004). Noncommunicable diseases: Risk factors and regional strategies for prevention and care. *Eastern Mediterranean Health Journal, 10*(6), 778–788.

Kim, Y., Yoo, K. Y., & Goodman, M. T. (2015). Differences in incidence, mortality and survival of breast cancer by regions and countries in Asia and contributing factors. *Asian Pacific Journal of Cancer Prevention, 16*(7), 2857–2870.

Kirwan, J. P., Sacks, J., & Nieuwoudt, S. (2017). The essential role of exercise in the management of type 2 diabetes. *Cleveland Clinic Journal of Medicine, 84*(7 Suppl 1), S15.

Klein, W. M., Jacobsen, P. B., & Helzlsouer, K. J. (2020). Alcohol and cancer risk: Clinical and research implications. *JAMA, 323*(1), 23–24.

Krutz, M., Acharya, P., Chissoe, G., Raj, V., Driskill, L., Krempl, G., et al. (2022). Tobacco cessation after head and neck cancer diagnosis is an independent predictor of treatment response and long-term survival. *Oral Oncology, 134*, 106072.

Kuan, A. S., Green, J., Kitahara, C. M., De González, A. B., Key, T., K. Reeves, G., et al. (2019). Diet and risk of glioma: Combined analysis of 3 large prospective studies in the UK and USA. *Neuro-Oncology, 21*(7), 944–952.

Kumar, A., Chinnathambi, S., Kumar, M., & Pandian, G. N. (2023). Food intake and colorectal cancer. *Nutrition and Cancer, 75*(9), 1710–1742.

Lăcătuşu, C. M., Grigorescu, E. D., Floria, M., Onofriescu, A., & Mihai, B. M. (2019). The Mediterranean diet: From an environment-driven food culture to an emerging medical prescription. *International Journal of Environmental Research and Public Health, 16*(6), 942.

Lei, X., Song, S., Li, X., Geng, C., & Wang, C. (2021). Excessive body fat at a young age increases the risk of colorectal cancer: A systematic review and meta-analysis. *Nutrition and Cancer, 73*(9), 1601–1612.

Leiter, A., Veluswamy, R. R., & Wisnivesky, J. P. (2023). The global burden of lung cancer: Current status and future trends. *Nature Reviews Clinical Oncology, 20*(9), 624–639.

Li, Y., Pan, A., Wang, D. D., Liu, X., Dhana, K., Franco, O. H., et al. (2018). Impact of healthy lifestyle factors on life expectancies in the US population. *Circulation, 138*(4), 345–355.

Lin, X., & Li, H. (2021). Obesity: Epidemiology, pathophysiology, and therapeutics. *Frontiers in Endocrinology, 12*, 706978.

Ludwig, D. S., Peterson, K. E., & Gortmaker, S. L. (2001). Relation between consumption of sugar-sweetened drinks and childhood obesity: A prospective, observational analysis. *The Lancet, 357*(9255), 505–508.

Maiuolo, J., Gliozzi, M., Carresi, C., Musolino, V., Oppedisano, F., Scarano, F., et al. (2021). Nutraceuticals and cancer: Potential for natural polyphenols. *Nutrients, 13*(11), 3834.

Mandic, M., Safizadeh, F., Niedermaier, T., Hoffmeister, M., & Brenner, H. (2023). Association of overweight, obesity, and recent weight loss with colorectal cancer risk. *JAMA Network Open, 6*(4), e239556.

Marino, P., Pepe, G., Basilicata, M. G., Vestuto, V., Marzocco, S., Autore, G., et al. (2023). Potential role of natural antioxidant products in oncological diseases. *Antioxidants, 12*(3), 704.

McNabb, S., Harrison, T. A., Albanes, D., Berndt, S. I., Brenner, H., Caan, B. J., et al. (2020). Meta-analysis of 16 studies of the association of alcohol with colorectal cancer. *International Journal of Cancer, 146*(3), 861–873.
McTiernan, A. N. N. E., Friedenreich, C. M., Katzmarzyk, P. T., Powell, K. E., Macko, R., Buchner, D., et al. (2019). Physical activity in cancer prevention and survival: A systematic review. *Medicine and Science in Sports and Exercise, 51*(6), 1252.
McTiernan, A., Kooperberg, C., White, E., Wilcox, S., Coates, R., Adams-Campbell, L. L., et al. (2004). Recreational physical activity and the risk of breast cancer in postmenopausal women: The women's health initiative cohort study. *Obstetrical & Gynecological Survey, 59*(3), 203–204.
Miller, E. R., Wilson, C., Chapman, J., Flight, I., Nguyen, A. M., Fletcher, C., & Ramsey, I. (2018). Connecting the dots between breast cancer, obesity and alcohol consumption in middle-aged women: Ecological and case control studies. *BMC Public Health, 18*, 1–14.
Morze, J., Danielewicz, A., Przybyłowicz, K., Zeng, H., Hoffmann, G., & Schwingshackl, L. (2021). An updated systematic review and meta-analysis on adherence to mediterranean diet and risk of cancer. *European Journal of Nutrition, 60*, 1561–1586.
Muffone, A. R. M., de Oliveira Lübke, P. D., & Rabito, E. I. (2023). Mediterranean diet and infertility: A systematic review with meta-analysis of cohort studies. *Nutrition Reviews, 81*(7), 775–789.
Nanri, A., Mizoue, T., Noda, M., Takahashi, Y., Kato, M., Inoue, M., & Tsugane, S. (2010). Rice intake and type 2 diabetes in Japanese men and women: The Japan public health center–based prospective study. *The American Journal of Clinical Nutrition, 92*(6), 1468–1477.
Nseir, W., Nassar, F., & Assy, N. (2010). Soft drinks consumption and nonalcoholic fatty liver disease. *World Journal of Gastroenterology: WJG, 16*(21), 2579.
Pelser, C., Mondul, A. M., Hollenbeck, A. R., & Park, Y. (2013). Dietary fat, fatty acids, and risk of prostate cancer in the NIH-AARP diet and health study. *Cancer Epidemiology, Biomarkers & Prevention, 22*(4), 697–707.
Petrelli, F., Cortellini, A., Indini, A., Tomasello, G., Ghidini, M., Nigro, O., et al. (2021). Association of obesity with survival outcomes in patients with cancer: A systematic review and meta-analysis. *JAMA Network Open, 4*(3), e213520–e213520.
Platz, E. A., Willett, W. C., Colditz, G. A., Rimm, E. B., Spiegelman, D., & Giovannucci, E. (2000). Proportion of colon cancer risk that might be preventable in a cohort of middle-aged US men. *Cancer Causes & Control, 11*, 579–588.
Ratnani, S., & Malik, S. (2022). Therapeutic properties of green tea: A review. *Journal of Multidisciplinary Applied Natural Science, 2*(2), 90–102.
Rawla, P., Sunkara, T., & Barsouk, A. (2019). Epidemiology of colorectal cancer: Incidence, mortality, survival, and risk factors. *Gastroenterology Review/Przegląd Gastroenterologiczny, 14*(2), 89–103.
Rosner, B., Eliassen, A. H., Toriola, A. T., Chen, W. Y., Hankinson, S. E., Willett, W. C., et al. (2017). Weight and weight changes in early adulthood and later breast cancer risk. *International Journal of Cancer, 140*(9), 2003–2014.
Ruiz, R. B., & Hernández, P. S. (2014). Diet and cancer: Risk factors and epidemiological evidence. *Maturitas, 77*(3), 202–208.
Rumgay, H., Shield, K., Charvat, H., Ferrari, P., Sornpaisarn, B., Obot, I., et al. (2021). Global burden of cancer in 2020 attributable to alcohol consumption: A population-based study. *The Lancet Oncology, 22*(8), 1071–1080.
Sami, W., Ansari, T., Butt, N. S., & Ab Hamid, M. R. (2017). Effect of diet on type 2 diabetes mellitus: A review. *International Journal of Health Sciences, 11*(2), 65.
Sangrajrang, S., Chaiwerawattana, A., Ploysawang, P., Nooklang, K., Jamsri, P., & Somharnwong, S. (2013). Obesity, diet and physical inactivity and risk of breast cancer in Thai women. *Asian Pacific Journal of Cancer Prevention, 14*(11), 7023–7027.
Santos, L. (2022). The impact of nutrition and lifestyle modification on health. *European Journal of Internal Medicine, 97*, 18–25.

Scholz, C., Andergassen, U., Hepp, P., Schindlbeck, C., Friedl, T. W., Harbeck, N., et al. (2015). Obesity as an independent risk factor for decreased survival in node-positive high-risk breast cancer. *Breast Cancer Research and Treatment, 151*, 569–576.

Schwingshackl, L., Schwedhelm, C., Galbete, C., & Hoffmann, G. (2017). Adherence to Mediterranean diet and risk of cancer: An updated systematic review and meta-analysis. *Nutrients, 9*(10), 1063.

Shahid, R. K., Ahmed, S., Le, D., & Yadav, S. (2021). Diabetes and cancer: Risk, challenges, management and outcomes. *Cancers, 13*(22), 5735.

Sheikh, M., Mukeriya, A., Shangina, O., Brennan, P., & Zaridze, D. (2021). Postdiagnosis smoking cessation and reduced risk for lung cancer progression and mortality: A prospective cohort study. *Annals of Internal Medicine, 174*(9), 1232–1239.

Siegel, R. L., Miller, K. D., Wagle, N. S., & Jemal, A. (2023). Cancer statistics, 2023. *CA: a Cancer Journal for Clinicians, 73*(1), 17–48.

Smith, R. A., Andrews, K. S., Brooks, D., Fedewa, S. A., Manassaram-Baptiste, D., Saslow, D., & Wender, R. C. (2019). Cancer screening in the United States, 2019: A review of current American Cancer Society guidelines and current issues in cancer screening. *CA: a Cancer Journal for Clinicians, 69*(3), 184–210.

Snowling, N. J., & Hopkins, W. G. (2006). Effects of different modes of exercise training on glucose control and risk factors for complications in type 2 diabetic patients: A meta-analysis. *Diabetes Care, 29*(11), 2518–2527.

Solans, M., Castelló, A., Benavente, Y., Marcos-Gragera, R., Amiano, P., Gracia-Lavedan, E., et al. (2018). Adherence to the Western, Prudent, and Mediterranean dietary patterns and chronic lymphocytic leukemia in the MCC-Spain study. *Haematologica, 103*(11), 1881.

Spyrou, N., Avgerinos, K. I., Mantzoros, C. S., & Dalamaga, M. (2018). Classic and novel adipocytokines at the intersection of obesity and cancer: Diagnostic and therapeutic strategies. *Current Obesity Reports, 7*, 260–275.

Sung, H., Siegel, R. L., Torre, L. A., Pearson-Stuttard, J., Islami, F., Fedewa, S. A., et al. (2019). Global patterns in excess body weight and the associated cancer burden. *CA: a Cancer Journal for Clinicians, 69*(2), 88–112.

Taheri, S., Lin, L., Austin, D., Young, T., & Mignot, E. (2004). Short sleep duration is associated with reduced leptin, elevated ghrelin, and increased body mass index. *PLoS Medicine, 1*(3), e62.

Tzenios, N. (2023). Obesity as a risk factor for different types of cancer. *EPRA International Journal of Research and Development (IJRD), 8*(2), 97–100.

Ugai, T., Sasamoto, N., Lee, H. Y., Ando, M., Song, M., Tamimi, R. M., et al. (2022). Is early-onset cancer an emerging global epidemic? Current evidence and future implications. *Nature Reviews Clinical Oncology, 19*(10), 656–673.

Van Blarigan, E. L., Fuchs, C. S., Niedzwiecki, D., Zhang, S., Saltz, L. B., Mayer, R. J., et al. (2018). Association of survival with adherence to the American Cancer Society nutrition and physical activity guidelines for cancer survivors after colon cancer diagnosis: The CALGB 89803/alliance trial. *JAMA Oncology, 4*(6), 783–790.

van den Brandt, P. A., Ziegler, R. G., Wang, M., Hou, T., Li, R., Adami, H. O., et al. (2021). Body size and weight change over adulthood and risk of breast cancer by menopausal and hormone receptor status: A pooled analysis of 20 prospective cohort studies. *European Journal of Epidemiology, 36*, 37–55.

Vasanth, R., Ganesh, A., & Shanker, R. (2017). Impact of stress on type 2 diabetes mellitus management. *Psychiatria Danubina, 29*(suppl. 3), 416–421.

Ventriglio, A., Sancassiani, F., Contu, M. P., Latorre, M., Di Salvatore, M., Fornaro, M., & Bhugra, D. (2020). Mediterranean diet and its benefits on health and mental health: A literature review. *Clinical Practice and Epidemiology in Mental Health: CP & EMH, 16*(Suppl-1), 156.

Vgontzas, A. N., Liao, D., Pejovic, S., Calhoun, S., Karataraki, M., & Bixler, E. O. (2009). Insomnia with objective short sleep duration is associated with type 2 diabetes: A population-based study. *Diabetes Care, 32*(11), 1980–1985.

Villegas, R., Shu, X. O., Gao, Y. T., Yang, G., Elasy, T., Li, H., & Zheng, W. (2008). Vegetable but not fruit consumption reduces the risk of type 2 diabetes in Chinese women. *The Journal of Nutrition, 138*(3), 574–580.

Vineis, P., & Wild, C. P. (2014). Global cancer patterns: Causes and prevention. *The Lancet, 383*(9916), 549–557.

Wang, Q., & Zhou, W. (2021). Roles and molecular mechanisms of physical exercise in cancer prevention and treatment. *Journal of Sport and Health Science, 10*(2), 201–210.

Włodarczyk, M., & Nowicka, G. (2019). Obesity, DNA damage, and development of obesity-related diseases. *International Journal of Molecular Sciences, 20*(5), 1146.

Xie, F., You, Y., Huang, J., Guan, C., Chen, Z., Fang, M., et al. (2021). Association between physical activity and digestive-system cancer: An updated systematic review and meta-analysis. *Journal of Sport and Health Science, 10*(1), 4–13.

Youn, H. J., & Han, W. (2020). A review of the epidemiology of breast cancer in Asia: Focus on risk factors. *Asian Pacific Journal of Cancer Prevention: APJCP, 21*(4), 867.

Zhang, C., Cheng, Y., Luo, D., Wang, J., Liu, J., Luo, Y., et al. (2021). Association between cardiovascular risk factors and colorectal cancer: A systematic review and meta-analysis of prospective cohort studies. *EClinicalMedicine, 34, 100794.*

Zhang, D., Nichols, H. B., Troester, M., Cai, J., Bensen, J. T., & Sandler, D. P. (2020). Tea consumption and breast cancer risk in a cohort of women with family history of breast cancer. *International Journal of Cancer, 147*(3), 876–886.

The Importance of Understanding the Link Between Diabetes and Cancer

Chandramohan Kiruthiga, Mamali Das, Arumugam Kamaladevi, and K. Langeswaran

Abstract

The increasing global prevalence of diabetes and cancer presents a critical challenge for healthcare systems, as both conditions are driven by overlapping metabolic, environmental, and lifestyle factors. This chapter situates its discussion within the broader context of noncommunicable disease epidemiology, emphasizing that diabetes and cancer are not isolated disorders but interconnected pathophysiological entities sharing common biological mechanisms. It explores how the rising incidence of type 2 diabetes parallels the global escalation of cancer cases which is an epidemiological convergence largely attributed to obesity, sedentary lifestyles, aging populations, and nutritional transitions toward energy-dense diets. The chapter delineates the molecular, clinical, and societal dimensions of the diabetes–cancer relationship. It discusses the mechanistic underpinnings, including hyperinsulinemia, insulin-like growth factor signaling, chronic inflammation, oxidative stress, and dysregulated glucose metabolism that foster oncogenesis in diabetic milieus. Conversely, it examines how cancer therapies such as chemotherapy, radiotherapy, and corticosteroids aggravate insulin resistance, precipitating or worsening diabetes. The chapter also underscores the unique clinical vulnerabilities of diabetic cancer patients, including heightened toxicity, impaired recovery, and increased recurrence risks.

Further, the chapter presents preventive strategies encompassing lifestyle modification, metformin therapy, and evidence-based dietary interventions. It also follows on the transformative role of artificial intelligence, big data, and multi-omics technologies in predicting disease trajectories, identifying biomarkers, and enabling personalized care. The chapter of the book also emphasizes the ethical and public health imperatives, thus addressing healthcare inequities,

C. Kiruthiga · M. Das · A. Kamaladevi · K. Langeswaran (✉)
Department of Biomedical Science, Faculty of Science, Alagappa University, Karaikudi, TN, India

R. Noor (ed.), *Diabetes and Cancer: Association, Mechanism, and Therapeutic Implications*, https://doi.org/10.1007/978-981-95-5651-9_6

expanding access to screening and education, and implementing cost-effective interventions, particularly in low- and middle-income countries.

Toward the end, this chapter provides a holistic framework for understanding how diabetes and cancer converge at the molecular, clinical, and policy levels. By integrating biomedical evidence with population-level strategies, it advocates a shift from disease-specific management toward a unified, prevention-oriented paradigm capable of reducing the global burden of both disorders and fostering equitable, sustainable health outcomes.

Keywords

Insulin resistance · Hyperinsulinemia · Chronic inflammation · Oxidative stress · Metabolic reprogramming · Insulin-like growth factor-1 (IGF-1) · Metformin therapy · Precision medicine

Diabetes and cancer are significant global health concerns, both of which are linked to increased mortality and morbidity rates. Common risk factors, such as obesity, age, and sedentary behavior, as well as fundamental biological processes like insulin resistance, chronic inflammation, and hyperglycemia, influence the intricate interaction among a variety of chronic illnesses. It is imperative to comprehend the relationship between diabetes and cancer to facilitate early detection, risk mitigation, and effective care treatment. Patients with diabetes have an elevated risk of developing a variety of malignancies, such as pancreatic, liver, colorectal, breast, and endometrial tumors, as evident in numerous epidemiological studies. This increased susceptibility is attributed to hyperinsulinemia, oxidative stress, and proinflammatory cytokine activity, all of which promote carcinogenesis. Cancer survivors who have diabetes experience unique challenges in terms of treatment outcomes, as diabetes can exacerbate the toxicity of chemotherapy, impede surgical recuperation, and increase the likelihood of cardiovascular events.

In order to address these dual health challenges, it is imperative to implement a comprehensive approach that includes lifestyle modifications, personalized diagnostic procedures, and specific pharmaceutical therapies. The function of antidiabetic medications, particularly metformin, in modifying the risk of cancer is a topic of ongoing research, with promising results suggesting that they have the potential to impede the proliferation of tumors. Moreover, in order to reduce the incidence of these maladies, public health campaigns should prioritize preventative strategies, including the promotion of physical activity, nutritious diets, and smoking cessation. The focus of future research should be on the identification of biomarkers for early diagnosis, the investigation of precision medicine strategies, and the clarification of the molecular mechanisms that connect diabetes and cancer. Healthcare systems have the potential to enhance patient outcomes and reduce the global burden of diabetes and cancer by encouraging multidisciplinary collaboration among oncologists, endocrinologists, and primary care clinicians. To improve the quality of life for those affected by these disorders, it is essential to establish more effective preventative and treatment measures through collaboration among academicians, healthcare practitioners, and policymakers.

1 Summarizing the Relationship Between Diabetes and Cancer

The bidirectional relationship between diabetes and cancer is emphasized by the evidence presented in chapters "An Overview of Diabetes and Cancer Risks: Types and Mechanisms" and "Understanding the Connection Between Diabetes and Cancer". An elevated risk of developing specific varieties of cancer, such as liver, pancreatic, endometrial, colorectal, and breast cancer, is associated with diabetes, particularly type 2 diabetes (Giovannucci et al., 2010; Vigneri et al., 2009). On the other hand, metabolic dysfunction can be exacerbated by cancer and its treatments, resulting in the onset or exacerbation of diabetes (Gallagher & LeRoith, 2011). The overlapping pathophysiology of these diseases is influenced by shared risk factors, including obesity, sedentary occupations, inadequate diet, and aging (Lauby-Secretan et al., 2016). Dysregulated glucose metabolism, chronic inflammation, and hyperinsulinemia are critical biological mechanisms that contribute to the diabetes–cancer relationship (Pollak, 2012).

Hyperinsulinemia plays a notably significant function in the development of cancer. Insulin is a hormone that promotes growth, and its elevated levels can promote the proliferation of cancer cells (Pollak, 2012). Insulin-like growth factor-1 (IGF-1), which is structurally similar to insulin, is also essential for the progression of cancer by promoting cell proliferation and inhibiting apoptosis (Gallagher & LeRoith, 2011). Chronic inflammation, which is a defining characteristic of both diabetes and cancer, exacerbates this relationship by establishing a microenvironment that promotes tumor growth (Greten & Grivennikov, 2019). Individuals with diabetes exhibit elevated levels of inflammatory cytokines, including TNF-α and IL-6, which have been linked to the development of cancer (Wu et al., 2016).

The influence of dysregulated glucose metabolism on the progression of cancer is impossible to ignore. The Warburg effect is a phenomenon in which cancer cells preferentially utilize glycolysis for energy production, even in the presence of oxygen (Chen et al., 2015). This metabolic reprogramming enables cancer cells to adapt to hypoxic conditions and proliferate swiftly. In individuals with diabetes, chronic hyperglycemia supplies an abundant supply of glucose, which in turn stimulates the proliferation of cancer cells (Schiliro & Firestein, 2021). Additionally, it has been demonstrated that advanced glycation end-products (AGEs), which accumulate in individuals with inadequately controlled diabetes, contribute to the progression of cancer by promoting oxidative stress and inflammation (Uribarri et al., 2015).

2 Clinical Consequences for Cancer Patients and Survivors

The distinctive obstacles encountered by cancer survivors with diabetes were emphasized in chapter "Diabetes in Cancer Survivors". A multidisciplinary approach that includes oncologists, endocrinologists, and healthcare providers is necessary to manage the dual burden of managing both conditions (Shahid et al., 2021). Close monitoring and customized interventions are required due to the potential impairment of glucose metabolism that can result from cancer treatments, such as chemotherapy and radiation (Hershey et al., 2012). Additionally, the necessity of integrated care models that simultaneously address both conditions is underscored by the fact that cancer survivors with diabetes are at a heightened risk of recurrence and mortality (Barone, 2008). Chemotherapy-induced hyperglycemia is a prevalent complication in cancer patients with diabetes. Insulin resistance can be exacerbated, and pancreatic β-cell function can be impaired by specific chemotherapeutic agents, including glucocorticoids and mTOR inhibitors (Shahid et al., 2021). Radiation therapy, particularly when directed at the pancreas or liver, can also disrupt glucose homeostasis by damaging insulin-producing cells or altering hepatic glucose metabolism (Jiang et al., 2020). These metabolic disturbances may persist for an extended period following the conclusion of cancer treatment, necessitating ongoing monitoring and management.

The effects of diabetes on cancer outcomes are well documented. Research has demonstrated that cancer patients with diabetes have a lower overall survival rate than their nondiabetic counterparts (Barone, 2008). This disparity is the result of a variety of factors, such as an increase in treatment-related complications, suboptimal treatment adherence, and delayed diagnosis (Hoagland & Kipping, 2024). Furthermore, diabetes is linked to an elevated risk of cancer recurrence, notably in hormone-sensitive malignancies like breast and prostate cancer (Giovannucci et al., 2010). These results emphasize the significance of incorporating diabetes management into cancer care to enhance outcomes and alleviate the disease's burden.

3 Risk Reduction Strategies

Chapter "Strategies for Reducing the Risk of Diabetes and Cancer" delineated evidence-based strategies for mitigating the risk of cancer and diabetes. Lifestyle modifications, including the adoption of a balanced diet that is rich in whole cereals, fruits, and vegetables, regular physical activity, and the maintenance of a healthy weight, are essential for prevention (Rippe, 2018). Pharmacological interventions, such as metformin for diabetes management, have demonstrated potential in reducing the risk of cancer; however, additional research is required to confirm their efficacy (DeCensi et al., 2010). It is imperative to implement public health initiatives that are designed to reduce the impact of both conditions on individuals and healthcare systems by increasing awareness and promoting early screening (Siegel et al., 2020). The significance of diet in the prevention of cancer and diabetes is not overstated. The risk of both conditions has been demonstrated to be reduced by the

Mediterranean diet, which is defined by its high consumption of fruits, vegetables, whole cereals, and healthful fats (Martín-Peláez et al., 2020). This dietary pattern is abundant in anti-inflammatory compounds and antioxidants, which mitigate oxidative stress and inflammation, which are critical factors in the development of cancer and diabetes (Weinberg Sibony et al., 2024). In contrast, a diet that is rich in processed meats, refined carbohydrates, and saturated fats is linked to an elevated risk of cancer and diabetes (Qian et al., 2020).

Physical activity is an additional essential element in the prevention of cancer and diabetes. Insulin sensitivity is enhanced, systemic inflammation is diminished, and healthy weight maintenance is facilitated by consistent exercise (Chomiuk et al., 2024). Epidemiological studies have consistently shown that physically active individuals have a lower risk of developing diabetes and certain types of cancer, including breast, colorectal, and endometrial cancer (Kerr et al., 2017). These protective effects are mediated by enhanced immune function, reduced levels of circulating growth factors, and improved glucose metabolism (Hojman et al., 2018). Pharmacological interventions, particularly metformin, have garnered significant attention for their potential anticancer properties. Metformin, a first-line treatment for type 2 diabetes, has been shown to reduce cancer risk and improve outcomes in diabetic patients (DeCensi et al., 2010). Metformin's anticancer effects are achieved through a variety of mechanisms, such as the activation of AMP-activated protein kinase (AMPK), the inhibition of mTOR signaling, and the reduction of circulating insulin levels (Zi et al., 2017). Nevertheless, additional research is required to ascertain the most effective dosing, duration, and patient populations for the use of metformin in the prevention and treatment of cancer.

4 The Function of Research and Innovation

Although substantial progress has been achieved in comprehending the relationship between diabetes and cancer, numerous inquiries remain unresolved. The molecular mechanisms that underlie this connection should be the primary focus of future research, as well as the identification of biomarkers for early detection and the development of targeted therapies that address both conditions (Gallagher & LeRoith, 2011). To assess the efficacy of interventions and develop clinical guidelines, it is imperative to conduct extensive longitudinal studies and randomized controlled trials (Giovannucci et al., 2010). Furthermore, the utilization of big data analytics and artificial intelligence advancements could offer novel perspectives on personalized prevention and treatment strategies (Badr et al., 2024; Jiang et al., 2017). The development of biomarkers for early detection of diabetes and cancer is a promising area of research. Biomarkers such as circulating tumor DNA (ctDNA), microRNAs, and metabolic signatures have shown potential for identifying individuals at high risk of developing these conditions (Felekkis & Papaneophytou, 2024; Liu et al., 2024). Timely intervention is facilitated by early detection, which can substantially enhance outcomes and alleviate the burden of disease. In addition, the potential to disentangle the intricate interplay between metabolic and oncological pathways is demonstrated by the integration of multi-omics data, such as genomics, transcriptomics, and metabolomics (Arjmand et al., 2022; Qiu et al., 2023).

Artificial intelligence (AI) and machine learning are revolutionizing the field of diabetes and cancer research. These technologies enable the analysis of large datasets, identification of patterns, and prediction of disease outcomes with unprecedented accuracy (Jiang et al., 2017). For instance, AI-driven algorithms are being implemented to anticipate patient responses to chemotherapy, optimize insulin dosing in diabetic patients, and detect early indications of cancer in medical imaging. Ultimately, patient outcomes can be enhanced through the use of AI-driven algorithms, which can aid in risk stratification, early diagnosis, and personalized treatment planning (Guan et al., 2023). Nevertheless, the safe and effective implementation of AI in healthcare necessitates the resolution of the ethical and regulatory challenges (Mennella et al., 2024).

5 A Call to Action for Healthcare Providers and Policymakers

Healthcare providers are essential in addressing the diabetes–cancer connection. It is imperative that routine screening for diabetes in cancer patients and vice versa become standard practice. Healthcare professionals can improve their capacity to effectively manage these intricate comorbidities through education and training programs (Hershey et al., 2012). Policymakers must prioritize financing for public health initiatives and research that are designed to alleviate the burden of cancer and diabetes (Siegel et al., 2020). To establish a healthcare ecosystem that promotes prevention, early detection, and comprehensive care, governments, healthcare organizations, and advocacy groups must collaborate.

A paradigm transformation in healthcare delivery is necessary to integrate diabetes and cancer care. The complex requirements of patients with both conditions necessitate the collaboration of multidisciplinary teams, which include oncologists, endocrinologists, dietitians, and primary care providers. Patient-centered care models that prioritize individualized treatment plans and shared decision-making can improve outcomes and enhance patient satisfaction (Barry & Edgman-Levitan, 2012). Additionally, remote monitoring and administration can be facilitated by the use of digital health tools and telemedicine, particularly in marginalized populations (Haleem et al., 2021). To resolve the diabetes–cancer link, policymakers must assume a critical role. The development of evidence-based guidelines for prevention, screening, and management necessitates national and international collaborations. It is imperative to implement public health initiatives that are designed to decrease the prevalence of obesity, which is a significant risk factor for both cancer and diabetes (Lauby-Secretan et al., 2016). Furthermore, the burden of these diseases can be substantially diminished by policies that encourage the development of healthier dietary environments, increased physical activity, and early screening for metabolic and oncological conditions (Siegel et al., 2020).

6 Addressing Health Disparities and Access to Care

Health disparities, particularly in underserved populations worldwide, have a substantial impact on the relationship between diabetes and cancer. Limited access to healthcare, socioeconomic challenges, and systemic inequities frequently result in these populations experiencing elevated rates of both conditions. For instance, the prevalence of diabetes and specific cancers, such as liver and cervical cancer, is disproportionately high in low- and middle-income countries (LMICs) as a result of deficient healthcare infrastructure, poverty, and inadequate education (International Diabetes Federation, 2021). These disparities are further exacerbated by barriers to early detection and treatment, including financial constraints, geographic isolation, and cultural stigmas. For instance, in sub-Saharan Africa, late-stage cancer diagnoses are prevalent as a result of inadequate healthcare resources and screening programs (Tfayli et al., 2010). In South Asia, the dual burden of diabetes and cancer is increasing, and there are substantial disparities in access to preventive care and treatment (Khan et al., 2019).

Targeted interventions are indispensable to rectify these disparities. These include the implementation of culturally sensitive outreach initiatives to foster early screening and build trust, the expansion of access to affordable healthcare services, particularly in rural and low-income regions, and the increase in funding for community health programs that provide education, screening, and preventive care (Braveman et al., 2018). For instance, telemedicine and mobile health clinics have demonstrated the potential to enhance access to care in Africa and India's remote regions (McGowan et al., 2020). Healthcare systems can alleviate the burden of diabetes and cancer in vulnerable populations and enhance global health outcomes by addressing these disparities.

7 Economic Impact and Cost-Effective Interventions

The economic burden of managing diabetes and cancer is significant, as both conditions contribute to high healthcare costs, reduced productivity, and a diminished quality of life. Globally, the annual cost of diabetes care is estimated at 760 billion, while cancer care costs are projected to exceed 458 billion by 2030 (International Diabetes Federation, 2021; Global Burden of Disease Collaborative Network, 2020). Cost-effective interventions are essential in LMICs, as they encounter an additional challenge as a result of their limited infrastructure and resources.

A cost-effective strategy that has been demonstrated to reduce the risk of both diabetes and cancer is the promotion of lifestyle modifications, such as increased physical activity and healthier nutrition (Piras & Raffi, 2023). For instance, community-based initiatives in Mexico and Brazil have effectively promoted healthier dietary practices and consistent physical activity, resulting in quantifiable enhancements in population health (Shirvani et al., 2021). This is an additional cost-effective strategy: investing in early detection programs. For example, cervical cancer screening programs in Thailand and breast cancer screening initiatives in India have shown substantial reductions in late-stage diagnoses and treatment costs (Martinez et al., 2024). Furthermore, the economic burden can be further alleviated by increasing the use of low-cost medications such as metformin, which has demonstrated the potential to reduce the risk of cancer in diabetic patients (DeCensi et al., 2010). Healthcare systems can enhance patient outcomes and alleviate the financial burden of diabetes and cancer by prioritizing these interventions.

8 Increasing Awareness to Empower Individuals

It is imperative to equip individuals with information regarding the relationship between diabetes and cancer to facilitate early intervention and prevention. Public awareness campaigns can be instrumental in educating individuals about the significance of lifestyle changes and shared risk factors. For instance, the World Health Organization's global campaigns on diabetes and cancer prevention have increased awareness in LMICs, promoting healthier behaviors and regularly scheduled screenings. Patient education is a fundamental component of prevention. Motivating individuals to adopt healthier lifestyles can be achieved by providing them with information regarding modifiable risk factors, including obesity, physical inactivity, and inadequate diet. Research has demonstrated that educational initiatives that offer practical methods for self-management, such as those implemented in Indonesia and South Africa, are effective in mitigating the risk factors associated with diabetes and cancer (Ernawati et al., 2021).

Patient engagement and adherence to preventive measures are being improved through the use of digital health platforms, such as mobile applications and online resources. For example, mobile health initiatives in developing countries have enhanced access to health information and promoted behavior change (Eze et al., 2018). Community-based interventions, including programs that encourage the cessation of smoking, physical activity, and healthy diets, have also been shown to be effective in decreasing the incidence of cancer and diabetes (Siegel et al., 2020). Supportive environments that promote healthy behaviors can be established through collaborative endeavors among healthcare organizations, schools, workplaces, and community centers.

9 Future Directions and Emerging Technologies

Future research should concentrate on precision medicine strategies that customize treatments according to an individual's genetic, metabolic, and oncological profile. Another promising area is the development of new biomarkers for early detection, such as circulating tumor DNA (ctDNA) and microRNAs. For instance, research conducted in China has identified specific microRNAs that are linked to both diabetes and cancer, which has the potential to develop targeted therapies and early diagnosis. Emerging evidence indicates that diabetes may affect the immune response to cancer, which is why immunotherapy is also garnering attention. Immunotherapy optimization for diabetic cancer patients is presently being investigated in Japan and Europe. Furthermore, the potential for real-time intervention and personalized care is demonstrated by advancements in ubiquitous technology, including continuous glucose monitors and devices that detect early cancer indicators. By investing in these regions, new opportunities for the prevention and treatment of cancer and diabetes can be unlocked, thereby enhancing global health outcomes.

To provide a comprehensive overview of the present understanding and future directions in diabetes–cancer research and treatment, Table 1 synthesizes the key aspects discussed throughout this chapter, including risk factors, biological mechanisms, prevention strategies, and emerging technologies. This synthesis serves as a foundation for future research priorities and clinical applications

Table 1 Comprehensive overview of the diabetes–cancer relationship

Aspect	Key points	Clinical implications
Shared risk factors	Obesity and metabolic syndrome Advanced age Physical inactivity Poor dietary patterns Tobacco use	BMI >30 increases cancer risk by 1.5–3.5 times Each 5 kg/m^2 increase in BMI raises cancer mortality by 10% Physical inactivity accounts for 9% of premature mortality
Biological mechanisms	Hyperinsulinemia and insulin resistance Chronic systemic inflammation Dysregulated glucose metabolism Oxidative stress Advanced glycation end-products (AGEs) • mTOR pathway activation	Insulin levels >25 μIU/mL associated with two times cancer risk Inflammatory markers IL-6 and TNF-α elevated two- to fourfold HbA1c >7.5% correlates with 1.8 times cancer risk ROS levels increased two to three times in diabetic patients
Associated cancer types	Pancreatic cancer (hazard ratio [HR]: 2.22) Hepatocellular carcinoma (HR: 2.50) Colorectal cancer (HR: 1.30) Breast cancer (HR: 1.20) Endometrial cancer (HR: 2.10) Bladder cancer (HR: 1.35)	Risk increases with diabetes duration Glycemic control impacts cancer progression Synergistic effect of obesity
Prevention strategies	Mediterranean diet adherence 150–300 min/week exercise 5–10% weight reduction target Smoking cessation programs Metformin therapy Regular cancer screening	Mediterranean diet reduces risk by 23% Exercise decreases cancer risk by 30–40% Metformin users show 31% lower cancer incidence Combined interventions show additive benefits

(continued)

Table 1 (continued)

Aspect	Key points	Clinical implications
Emerging technologies	AI-driven risk prediction models Multimodal machine learning Metabolomic biomarkers CGM with cancer detection Digital health integration	AI models achieve 94% sensitivity Machine learning reduces false positives by 45% Novel biomarkers improve early detection by 60% Real-time monitoring enables rapid intervention
Health disparities	Racial/ethnic disparities Socioeconomic factors Healthcare access barriers Cultural competency gaps Geographic variations	2.3 times higher mortality in underserved populations 45% lower screening rates in rural areas 60% higher cost burden in low-income groups
Research priorities	Molecular pathway studies Biomarker validation Clinical intervention trials Implementation research Population-specific studies	NIH funding priority area Multicenter trial initiatives Focus on precision medicine approaches Emphasis on translational outcomes

References

Arjmand, B., Hamidpour, S. K., Tayanloo-Beik, A., Goodarzi, P., Aghayan, H. R., Adibi, H., & Larijani, B. (2022). Machine learning: A new Prospect in multi-omics data analysis of cancer. *Frontiers in Genetics, 13*. https://doi.org/10.3389/fgene.2022.824451

Badr, Y., Abdul Kader, L., & Shamayleh, A. (2024). The use of big data in personalized healthcare to reduce inventory waste and optimize patient treatment. *Journal of Personalized Medicine, 14*. https://doi.org/10.3390/jpm14040383

Barone, B. B. (2008). Long-term all-cause mortality in cancer patients with preexisting diabetes mellitus. *JAMA, 300*, 2754. https://doi.org/10.1001/jama.2008.824

Barry, M. J., & Edgman-Levitan, S. (2012). Shared decision making — The pinnacle of patient-centered care. *The New England Journal of Medicine, 366*, 780–781. https://doi.org/10.1056/NEJMp1109283

Braveman, P., Arkin, E., Orleans, T., Proctor, D., Acker, J., & Plough, A. (2018). What is health equity? *Behavioral Science and Policy, 4*, 1–14. https://doi.org/10.1177/237946151800400102

Chen, X., Qian, Y., & Wu, S. (2015). The Warburg effect: Evolving interpretations of an established concept. *Free Radical Biology & Medicine, 79*, 253–263. https://doi.org/10.1016/j.freeradbiomed.2014.08.027

Chomiuk, T., Niezgoda, N., Mamcarz, A., & Śliż, D. (2024). Physical activity in metabolic syndrome. *Frontiers in Physiology, 15*. https://doi.org/10.3389/fphys.2024.1365761

DeCensi, A., Puntoni, M., Goodwin, P., Cazzaniga, M., Gennari, A., Bonanni, B., & Gandini, S. (2010). Metformin and cancer risk in diabetic patients: A systematic review and meta-analysis. *Cancer Prevention Research, 3*, 1451–1461. https://doi.org/10.1158/1940-6207.CAPR-10-0157

Ernawati, U., Wihastuti, T. A., & Utami, Y. W. (2021). Effectiveness of diabetes self-management education (DSME) in type 2 diabetes mellitus (T2DM) patients: Systematic literature review. *Journal of Public Health Research, 10*. https://doi.org/10.4081/jphr.2021.2240

Eze, E., Gleasure, R., & Heavin, C. (2018). Mobile health solutions in developing countries: A stakeholder perspective. *Health Systems (Basingstoke, England), 9*, 179–201. https://doi.org/10.1080/20476965.2018.1457134

Felekkis, K., & Papaneophytou, C. (2024). The circulating biomarkers league: Combining miRNAs with cell-free DNAs and proteins. *International Journal of Molecular Sciences, 25*, 3403. https://doi.org/10.3390/ijms25063403

Gallagher, E. J., & LeRoith, D. (2011). Diabetes, cancer, and metformin: Connections of metabolism and cell proliferation. *Annals of the New York Academy of Sciences, 1243*, 54–68. https://doi.org/10.1111/j.1749-6632.2011.06285.x

Giovannucci, E., Harlan, D. M., Archer, M. C., Bergenstal, R. M., Gapstur, S. M., Habel, L. A., Pollak, M., Regensteiner, J. G., & Yee, D. (2010). Diabetes and cancer. *Diabetes Care, 33*, 1674–1685. https://doi.org/10.2337/dc10-0666

Global Burden of Disease Collaborative Network, 2020. Global Burden of Disease Study 2019 (GBD 2019) Results.Institute for Health Metrics and Evaluation (IHME), Seattle, United States. Available from:http://ghdx.healthdata.org/gbd-results-tool

Greten, F. R., & Grivennikov, S. I. (2019). Inflammation and cancer: Triggers, mechanisms, and consequences. *Immunity, 51*, 27–41. https://doi.org/10.1016/j.immuni.2019.06.025

Guan, Z., Li, H., Liu, R., Cai, C., Liu, Y., Li, J., Wang, X., Huang, S., Wu, L., Liu, D., Yu, S., Wang, Z., Shu, J., Hou, X., Yang, X., Jia, W., & Sheng, B. (2023). Artificial intelligence in diabetes management: Advancements, opportunities, and challenges. *Cell Reports Medicine, 4*, 101213. https://doi.org/10.1016/j.xcrm.2023.101213

Haleem, A., Javaid, M., Singh, R. P., & Suman, R. (2021). Telemedicine for healthcare: Capabilities, features, barriers, and applications. *Sensors International, 2*, 100117. https://doi.org/10.1016/j.sintl.2021.100117

Hershey, D. S., Given, B., Given, C., Von Eye, A., & You, M. (2012). Diabetes and cancer: Impact on health-related quality of life. *Oncology Nursing Forum, 39*, 449–457. https://doi.org/10.1188/12.ONF.449-457

Hoagland, A., & Kipping, S. (2024). Challenges in promoting health equity and reducing disparities in access across new and established technologies. *The Canadian Journal of Cardiology, 40*, 1154–1167. https://doi.org/10.1016/j.cjca.2024.02.014

Hojman, P., Gehl, J., Christensen, J. F., & Pedersen, B. K. (2018). Molecular mechanisms linking exercise to cancer prevention and treatment. *Cell Metabolism, 27*, 10–21. https://doi.org/10.1016/j.cmet.2017.09.015

International Diabetes Federation, 2021. IDF Diabetes Atlas, 10th edn. International Diabetes Federation, Brussels, Belgium. Available from: https://diabetesatlas.org/

Jiang, F., Jiang, Y., Zhi, H., Dong, Y., Li, H., Ma, S., Wang, Y., Dong, Q., Shen, H., & Wang, Y. (2017). Artificial intelligence in healthcare: Past, present and future. *Stroke and Vascular Neurology, 2*, 230–243. https://doi.org/10.1136/svn-2017-000101

Jiang, S., Young, J. L., Wang, K., Qian, Y., & Cai, L. (2020). Diabetic-induced alterations in hepatic glucose and lipid metabolism: The role of type 1 and type 2 diabetes mellitus (Review). *Molecular Medicine Reports, 22*, 603–611. https://doi.org/10.3892/mmr.2020.11175

Kerr, J., Anderson, C., & Lippman, S. M. (2017). Physical activity, sedentary behaviour, diet, and cancer: An update and emerging new evidence. *The Lancet Oncology, 18*, e457–e471. https://doi.org/10.1016/S1470-2045(17)30411-4

Khan, M. A. B., Hashim, M. J., King, J. K., Govender, R. D., Mustafa, H., & Al Kaabi, J. (2019). Epidemiology of type 2 diabetes—Global burden of disease and forecasted trends. *Journal of Epidemiology and Global Health, 10*, 107. https://doi.org/10.2991/jegh.k.191028.001

Lauby-Secretan, B., Scoccianti, C., Loomis, D., Grosse, Y., Bianchini, F., & Straif, K. (2016). Body fatness and cancer — Viewpoint of the IARC working group. *The New England Journal of Medicine, 375*, 794–798. https://doi.org/10.1056/NEJMsr1606602

Liu, Z., Zhou, Y., Lu, J., Gong, T., Ibáñez, E., Cifuentes, A., & Lu, W. (2024). Microfluidic biosensors for biomarker detection in body fluids: A key approach for early cancer diagnosis. *Biomarker Research, 12*, 153. https://doi.org/10.1186/s40364-024-00697-4

Martín-Peláez, S., Fito, M., & Castaner, O. (2020). Mediterranean diet effects on type 2 diabetes prevention, disease progression, and related mechanisms. A Review. *Nutrients, 12*, 2236. https://doi.org/10.3390/nu12082236

Martinez, M. E., Schmeler, K. M., Lajous, M., & Newman, L. A. (2024). Cancer screening in low- and middle-income countries. *American Society of Clinical Oncology Educational Book, 44*. https://doi.org/10.1200/EDBK_431272

McGowan, C. R., Baxter, L., Deola, C., Gayford, M., Marston, C., Cummings, R., & Checchi, F. (2020). Mobile clinics in humanitarian emergencies: A systematic review. *Conflict and Health, 14*, 4. https://doi.org/10.1186/s13031-020-0251-8

Mennella, C., Maniscalco, U., De Pietro, G., & Esposito, M. (2024). Ethical and regulatory challenges of AI technologies in healthcare: A narrative review. *Heliyon, 10*, e26297. https://doi.org/10.1016/j.heliyon.2024.e26297

Piras, A., & Raffi, M. (2023). A narrative literature review on the role of exercise training in managing type 1 and type 2 diabetes mellitus. *Healthcare, 11*, 2947. https://doi.org/10.3390/healthcare11222947

Pollak, M. (2012). The insulin and insulin-like growth factor receptor family in neoplasia: An update. *Nature Reviews. Cancer, 12*, 159–169. https://doi.org/10.1038/nrc3215

Qian, F., Riddle, M. C., Wylie-Rosett, J., & Hu, F. B. (2020). Red and processed meats and health risks: How strong is the evidence? *Diabetes Care, 43*, 265–271. https://doi.org/10.2337/dci19-0063

Qiu, S., Cai, Y., Yao, H., Lin, C., Xie, Y., Tang, S., & Zhang, A. (2023). Small molecule metabolites: Discovery of biomarkers and therapeutic targets. *Signal Transduction and Targeted Therapy, 8*, 132. https://doi.org/10.1038/s41392-023-01399-3

Rippe, J. M. (2018). Lifestyle medicine: The health promoting power of daily habits and practices. *American Journal of Lifestyle Medicine, 12*, 499–512. https://doi.org/10.1177/1559827618785554

Schiliro, C., & Firestein, B. L. (2021). Mechanisms of metabolic reprogramming in cancer cells supporting enhanced growth and proliferation. *Cells, 10*, 1056. https://doi.org/10.3390/cells10051056

Shahid, R. K., Ahmed, S., Le, D., & Yadav, S. (2021). Diabetes and cancer: Risk, challenges, management and outcomes. *Cancers (Basel), 13*, 5735. https://doi.org/10.3390/cancers13225735

Shirvani, T., Javadivala, Z., Azimi, S., Shaghaghi, A., Fathifar, Z., Devender Bhalla, H. D. R., Abdekhoda, M., & Nadrian, H. (2021). Community-based educational interventions for prevention of type II diabetes: A global systematic review and meta-analysis. *Systematic Reviews, 10*, 81. https://doi.org/10.1186/s13643-021-01619-3

Siegel, R. L., Miller, K. D., & Jemal, A. (2020). Cancer statistics, 2020. *CA: a Cancer Journal for Clinicians, 70*, 7–30. https://doi.org/10.3322/caac.21590

Tfayli, A., Temraz, S., Abou Mrad, R., & Shamseddine, A. (2010). Breast cancer in low- and middle-income countries: An emerging and challenging epidemic. *Journal of Oncology, 2010*, 1–5. https://doi.org/10.1155/2010/490631

Uribarri, J., del Castillo, M. D., de la Maza, M. P., Filip, R., Gugliucci, A., Luevano-Contreras, C., Macías-Cervantes, M. H., Markowicz Bastos, D. H., Medrano, A., Menini, T., Portero-Otin, M., Rojas, A., Sampaio, G. R., Wrobel, K., Wrobel, K., & Garay-Sevilla, M. E. (2015). Dietary advanced glycation end products and their role in health and disease. *Advances in Nutrition, 6*, 461–473. https://doi.org/10.3945/an.115.008433

Vigneri, P., Frasca, F., Sciacca, L., Pandini, G., & Vigneri, R. (2009). Diabetes and cancer. *Endocrine-Related Cancer, 16*, 1103–1123. https://doi.org/10.1677/ERC-09-0087

Weinberg Sibony, R., Segev, O., Dor, S., & Raz, I. (2024). Overview of oxidative stress and inflammation in diabetes. *Journal of Diabetes, 16*, e70014. https://doi.org/10.1111/1753-0407.70014

Wu, Y., Dong, Y., Liu, Y., & Vadgama, J. (2016). Diabetes-associated dysregulated cytokines and cancer. *Integrative Cancer Science and Therapeutics, 3*. https://doi.org/10.15761/ICST.1000173

Zi, F., Zi, H., Li, Y., He, J., Shi, Q., & Cai, Z. (2017). Metformin and cancer: An existing drug for cancer prevention and therapy (Review). *Oncology Letters*. https://doi.org/10.3892/ol.2017.7412

Exploring the Role of Gut Microbiota in Diabetes and Colorectal Cancer

Neeharika Sara Sennie, Sibin Nambidi, Ashiq Shibili P, Antara Banerjee, and Arunkumar Radhakrishnan

Abstract

The gut microbiota has been recognised as a key modulator of metabolic health, affecting glucose homeostasis, insulin sensitivity, and inflammation. Alterations in gut microbial community, or dysbiosis, have been implicated in the onset and progression of type 2 diabetes mellitus (T2DM). Emerging evidence also implicates gut microbiota imbalance in colorectal cancer (CRC) with a common pathogenic pathway through chronic inflammation, dysregulated immune responses, and metabolic endotoxemia. Therapeutic interventions of the gut microbiota, such as the administration of probiotics, prebiotics, synbiotics, and dietary changes in diabetes and CRC, provide promising strategies for individualised interventions that may enhance metabolic and oncologic benefits. The knowledge of these interconnected strategies provides new avenues for the prevention and management of diabetes and CRC. This chapter explores the intricate relationships between gut microbiota and glucose metabolism, while it also discusses the effects of dietary and lifestyle interventions, and assesses the contribution of microbiota-derived metabolites to diabetes pathophysiology. In addition, it also highlights the new evidence linking diabetes and CRC through dysregulation of gut microbes.

N. S. Sennie · S. Nambidi · A. S. P · A. Banerjee (✉)
Medical Biotechnology Lab, Faculty of Allied Health Sciences, Chettinad Hospital and Research Institute (CHRI), Chettinad Academy of Research and Education (CARE), Chennai, Tamilnadu, India
e-mail: antarabanerjee@care.edu.in

A. Radhakrishnan (✉)
Department of Pharmacology, Chettinad Hospital and Research Institute (CHRI), Chettinad Academy of Research and Education (CARE), Chennai, Tamil Nadu, India
e-mail: arunkumarr@care.edu.in

R. Noor (ed.), *Diabetes and Cancer: Association, Mechanism, and Therapeutic Implications*, https://doi.org/10.1007/978-981-95-5651-9_7

Keywords

Gut microbiota · Type 2 diabetes mellitus · Colorectal cancer · Glucose homeostasis · Chronic inflammation · Probiotics and prebiotics

1 Introduction

Diabetes mellitus (DM) has become a significant global health concern, as its prevalence is escalating due to lifestyle changes, ageing populations, and genetic susceptibility (Craciun et al., 2022; Ma et al., 2019). It is a chronic metabolic disease characterised by hyperglycaemia, an increase in blood sugar level brought in by a deficiency in the secretion or action of insulin. This metabolic condition is classified as type 1, type 2, and gestational diabetes (Ma et al., 2019; Banday et al., 2020). Type 1 diabetes (T1D) is an autoimmune disease, characterised by T-cell-mediated destruction of pancreatic β-cells, resulting in insulin deficiency and eventually leading to hyperglycaemia. Type 2 diabetes (T2D) constitutes the majority of cases and is characterised by two main insulin aberrations: insulin resistance and β-cell malfunction. T2D constitutes a higher number of cases when compared with the former category. Obesity can also lead to hyperglycaemia as it is associated with increased body fat and diabetes. Gestational diabetes mellitus can be defined as the onset of diabetes during pregnancy, especially during the second and third trimesters. There are other types of diabetes, such as MODY (maturity-onset diabetes of the young), NDM (neonatal diabetes mellitus), etc. (Banday et al., 2020). In 2019, the global prevalence of diabetes was approximately 9.3% and is projected to increase to 10.2% by 2030 and 10.9% by 2045, with higher rates observed in urban areas (10.8%) compared to rural regions (7.2%) (Saeedi et al., 2019). As reported by the IDF (International Diabetes Federation) in 2021, around 537 million people worldwide were living with diabetes, accounting for about 10.5% of the global population (Hossain et al., 2024). This springing prevalence of diabetes focuses on the importance of understanding and maintaining glucose homeostasis to prevent the disruptions that lead to this chronic metabolic disorder. Glucose homeostasis is essential for maintaining stable blood glucose levels, achieved through the coordinated actions of insulin, glucagon, and various metabolic organs, including the pancreas, liver, muscles, and adipose tissues (Rajan et al., 2024). Insulin, produced by pancreatic β-cells, enhances glucose uptake by tissues, stimulates glycogen synthesis in the liver and muscles, promotes lipid storage in adipose tissue, and inhibits gluconeogenesis and glycogen breakdown (Milionis et al., 2023). Conversely, glucagon, secreted by pancreatic α-cells during fasting or low glucose levels, stimulates hepatic glucose production to sustain blood sugar levels (Campbell & Drucker, 2015). Insulin resistance disrupts glucose homeostasis, triggering hyperinsulinemia, weight gain, and a vicious cycle of worsening resistance (Milionis et al., 2023). This dysregulation plays a key role in developing T2D, as pancreatic β-cells eventually fail to produce sufficient insulin to overcome resistance, resulting in chronic hyperglycaemia (Wu et al., 2020). Excess body weight, chronic inflammation, altered lipid metabolism, and intestinal dysbiosis further aggravate insulin resistance. The persistent metabolic abnormality in diabetes leads to complications, like a substantial public health burden. Therefore, maintaining glucose homeostasis is essential to preventing the progression of prediabetes and T2D and mitigating associated complications (Campbell & Drucker, 2015, Wu et al., 2020). Studies suggest that the gut microbiota plays a crucial role in metabolic regulation, particularly glucose metabolism, by modulating insulin sensitivity, inflammation, and energy balance (Ho et al., 2015). The gut microbiome is a complex ecosystem of microorganisms, primarily bacteria, residing in the gastrointestinal tract and plays a pivotal role in human health (Camilleri, 2019). Its influence extends beyond the gut through mechanisms like intestinal permeability regulation, often called 'leaky gut'. Disruption in microbiota balance, or dysbiosis, can increase intestinal permeability, enabling harmful microbes and their metabolites to enter systemic circulation (Shreiner et al., 2015). This systemic interaction can trigger widespread effects, contributing to autoimmune conditions (e.g. T1D, inflammatory bowel disease), psychiatric disorders (e.g. anxiety, depression), metabolic diseases (e.g. obesity, T2D), and even cancers like CRC and hepatocellular carcinoma. The gut microbiota's profound influence on immunological regulation, metabolic health, and the gut-brain axis emphasises its key role in stabilising overall systemic homeostasis and highlights its therapeutic potential in treating numerous diseases (Ramadevi & Meenakshi, 2023). In addition to its pivotal role in diabetes, gut microbiota dysbiosis has also been associated with CRC, a very prevalent type of cancer worldwide. Chronic low-grade inflammation, dysfunction of intestinal barrier function, and microbial metabolite imbalance have been identified as causing both diabetes mellitus and CRC (Thursby & Juge, 2017). When lipopolysaccharides (LPS) and production of short-chain fatty acids (SCFA), the gut-derived substances, are affected, they induce insulin resistance, metabolic resistance, and tumorigenesis (Rinninella et al., 2019). This highlights the need to understand the interrelated functions of gut microbiota in both metabolic diseases, thereby noting its significance as a therapeutic target. This chapter reviews the crucial function of gut microbiota in metabolic control, highlighting its importance in glucose homeostasis and diabetes mellitus. It emphasises how dysbiosis of gut microbiota develops metabolic disease conditions such as T2D and CRC by causing chronic inflammation, disruption of intestinal barrier function, and shift in microbial metabolite production. These are interconnected pathways that impair insulin sensitivity and promote disease progression. The chapter also explores therapeutic strategies targeting the gut microbiota, including probiotics and prebiotics, aimed at maintaining metabolic balance and promoting clinical improvement in diabetic patients, emphasizing the gut microbiota as a promising target for managing diabetes and its complications.

2 Gut Microbiota Composition and Diversity

The human gastrointestinal tract accommodates 100 trillion microorganisms, home to a rich and varied microbial ecosystem, unevenly distributed along the gastrointestinal tract, with bacterial density increasing from the stomach (10 to 10^3 cells per gram) to the colon (10^{11} to 10^{12} cells per gram) (Bielka et al., 2022). The gut microbiome harbours a complex and dynamic microbiota (Fig. 1), a community of archaea, bacteria, and eukarya, co-evolved with the host (Rinninella et al., 2019). These microorganisms can significantly affect the physiology of individuals in both healthy and sick conditions. More than 1000 species of bacteria belonging to relatively few known phyla of bacteria, Bacteroidetes and Firmicutes, are the dominant ones, representing 90% of the gut microbiota. The phylum Firmicutes represents 90% of the phylum, followed by Bacteroidetes, Actinobacteria, Proteobacteria, Fusobacteria, and Verrucomicrobia (Vallianou et al., 2018). Firmicutes and Bacteroidetes play pivotal roles in energy extraction and metabolic processes. At the same time, Actinobacteria, such as *Bifidobacterium* species, contribute to intestinal health by producing short-chain fatty acids SCFAs like acetate, propionate, and butyrate. SCFAs regulate gut motility, enhance the intestinal barrier, and influence systemic functions, including insulin sensitivity and immune modulation (Sharlize

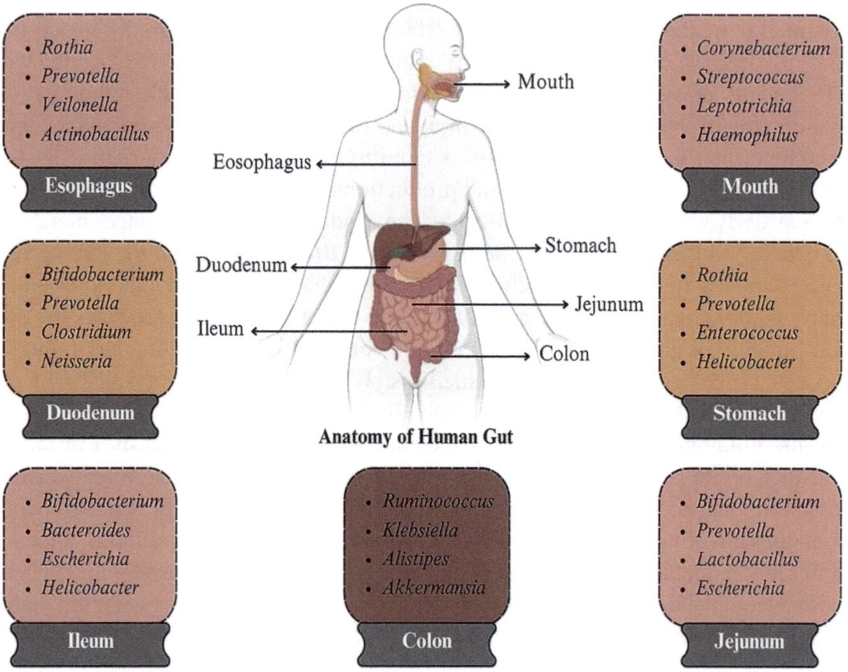

Fig. 1 Schematic representation of the human GIT highlighting the dominant bacterial genera at each anatomical site

Pedroza Matute & Sasitaran Iyavoo, 2023). Maintaining a balanced, diverse microbiota is crucial for sustaining gastrointestinal integrity, supporting the immune system, and preventing dysbiosis, which can lead to metabolic disorders like obesity, T2D, and other comorbidities (Sharlize Pedroza Matute & Sasitaran Iyavoo, 2023; Leeming et al., 2019). The gut microbiota performs diverse and critical functions necessary for the host's health, such as aiding digestion, synthesising vitamins (e.g. vitamin K and B-group vitamins), and producing SCFAs that regulate gut motility, strengthen the intestinal barrier, and improve glucose metabolism. It supports immune system development, protects against pathogen colonisation, and maintains metabolic functions, thereby maintaining gastrointestinal and systemic health (Vallianou et al., 2018). The composition and function of gut microbiota, as shown in Fig. 2, are determined by multiple factors, including diet, environment, geography, ethnicity, lifestyle choices, medicines, drugs, smoking, etc. (Leeming et al., 2019). Diet plays a pivotal role, with short- and long-term dietary patterns shaping microbial communities; high-fat, low-fibre diets are linked to *Bacteroides*-dominant profiles (Senghor et al., 2018). Geographic and ethnic variations reflect traditional diets and lifestyle habits. Rapid changes in microbiota occur with dietary changes, and migration to Western diets often reduces microbial diversity (Sbihi et al., 2019). Exposure to animal livestock and consumption of contaminated food, introduce varried microbial exposures that influence immune development and allergy risk and antibiotic resistance (Kumar et al., 2020). Antibiotics, environmental pollutants, and food additives cause dysbiosis. Lifestyle factors, including exercise, mental health, and circadian rhythms, also change the microbial diversity, with stress and sleep disruptions negatively impacting the gut health (Singh et al., 2022; Li et al., 2019; Cai et al., 2023; Frolova et al., 2022). These interconnected factors indicate

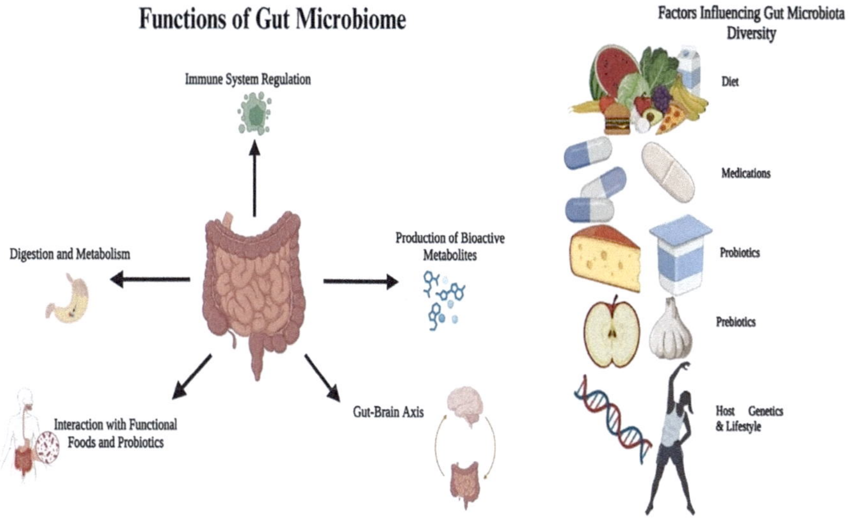

Fig. 2 Multifunctional roles of the gut microbiota and key factors affecting its composition, including diet, environment, genetics, medications, and lifestyle

the dynamic nature of the gut microbiome, adapting to external influences and shaping overall health.

3 Mechanisms of Microbiota in Glucose Homeostasis

3.1 Role of Short-Chain Fatty Acids in Insulin Resistance

SCFA are organic acids containing not more than six carbon atoms, predominantly generated in the colon through the fermentation of microbiota-accessible carbohydrates (MACs), such as dietary fibres (DF) and resistant starch (RS), by gut microbiota (Patloka et al., 2024). Key microbial contributors to SCFA production include species within the Firmicutes family, *Lachnospiraceae* and *Ruminococcaceae*, which ferment complex polysaccharides to generate butyrate, and *Bifidobacterium* species, which produce acetate from human milk oligosaccharides and other substrates (Martín et al., 2018). Among SCFAs, acetate accounts for approximately 60%, while propionate and butyrate contribute 20% each. Butyrate-producing bacteria, such as *Faecalibacterium prausnitzii*, are pivotal in maintaining gut health, supporting colonocyte energy needs, and preserving an anaerobic gut environment (Lange et al., 2023). SCFAs are rapidly taken up by colonic epithelial cells or transported into the systemic circulation, where they help in various metabolic processes, including lipid and glucose metabolism, highlighting their central role in host health (Martín et al., 2018; He et al., 2020). SCFAs play a crucial role in glucose homeostasis. They influence metabolism via mechanisms such as enhancing the expression of glucose transporter type 4 (GLUT4) and activating AMP-activated protein kinase (AMPK) pathways. At the cellular level, SCFAs increase the expression of GLUT4 in skeletal muscles, facilitating glucose transport into cells (Johanns et al., 2023). They also activate AMPK, a key energy sensor, by increasing the AMP/ATP ratio. In skeletal muscle, AMPK activation promotes glucose uptake and fatty acid oxidation while inhibiting glycogen synthesis. In the liver, AMPK is activated by butyrate and propionate, which suppresses gluconeogenesis by downregulating the expression of key enzymes like glucose-6-phosphatase (G6Pase) and phosphoenolpyruvate carboxykinase (PEPCK) which helps in the control of glucose level (Johanns et al., 2023; Yao et al., 2020). SCFAs stimulate the release of glucagon-like peptide-1 (GLP-1) by activating free fatty acid receptors (FFAR2) on colonic goblet cells, thereby enhancing insulin secretion and glucose tolerance. They also promote β-cell proliferation and gut-brain axis-mediated gluconeogenesis, improving glucose control and aiding weight loss (Mitoiu et al., 2024). Certain studies have found that changes in the composition of gut microbiota may enhance ghrelin (hunger hormone) levels or reduce the efficacy of satiety signals, potentially leading to overeating (Vigil et al., 2022; Nauck & Meier, 2018). SCFAs activate the G-coupled protein receptors, GPR41 and GPR43, stimulating the release of glucagon-like peptide-1 (GLP-1) and glucose-dependent insulinotropic peptide (GIP), also known as the incretin hormones, secreted by the gut in response to food, that are essential for regulating blood glucose levels after eating (Chia & Egan, 2019; El-Zayat et al.,

2019). Acetate regulates central appetite pathways and enhances lipid metabolism, while propionate supports hepatic gluconeogenesis and suppresses lipogenesis. They also interact with the gut-brain axis by modulating the neuroendocrine signalling, stress responses, and regulation of appetite, further supporting their influence on glucose homeostasis and energy balance (El-Zayat et al., 2019).

In addition to SCFAs, another crucial modulator is LPS. LPS greatly alter glucose metabolism by inducing systemic inflammation that results in the dysfunction of insulin signalling. LPS interacts with immune cells when moved into the bloodstream. When LPS bind to Toll-like receptor 4 (TLR4), they activate NF-κB and MAPK pathways, producing proinflammatory cytokines such as TNF-α, IL-6, and IL-1β. These cytokines dysregulate insulin receptor substrate (IRS) activity, lowering glucose uptake in peripheral tissues and thereby inducing insulin resistance (Xiao et al., 2018). Moreover, dietary patterns impact the activities of LPS, with one study demonstrating how a high-fat Western diet increased LPS activity and, therefore, glucose intolerance, while a fibre-rich diet, such as the Mediterranean diet, is associated with lower exposure to LPS and better glucose metabolism (Ahola et al., 2017; Suganya & Koo, 2020). The role of dietary fibre in gut microbiota-mediated metabolic control through SCFA production is represented in Fig. 3.

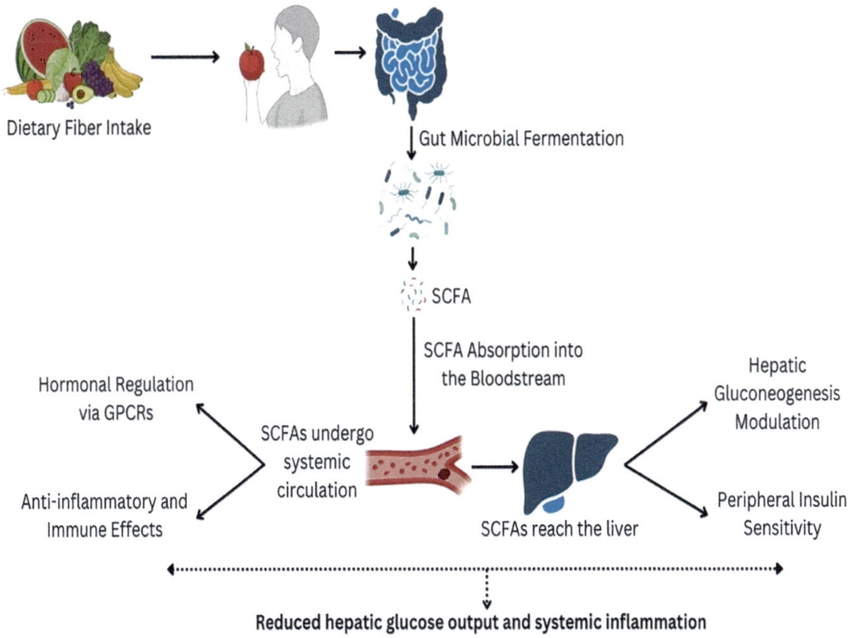

Fig. 3 Diagrammatic representation of dietary fibre fermentation by gut microbiota, leading to SCFA production, improved insulin sensitivity, hormonal regulation, and reduced glucose production for enhanced metabolic health

3.2 Gut-Brain Axis and Its Role in Glucose Regulation

The gut microbiota and gut-brain axis (GBA) are integral to each other, influencing neurodevelopment, neurotransmitter synthesis, and host stress responses through bidirectional communication pathways, essential for regulating physiological processes, including glucose homeostasis (Dash et al., 2022). These pathways include the autonomic nervous system (ANS) and the enteric nervous system (ENS), with the vagus nerve serving as a critical connection between the GIT and the brain (Nandwana et al., 2022; Breit et al., 2018). The vagus nerve modulates gut motility and immune responses. It transmits microbial signals to the brain, influencing neurotransmitter production, such as gamma-aminobutyric acid (GABA), serotonin, and SCFAs (McVey Neufeld et al., 2015). Studies have shown that germ-free (GF) mice (McVey Neufeld et al., 2012 2015) that lack microbiota exhibit reduced activation of ENS neurons and gut-brain signalling pathways, partly mediated by TLR4, which recognises LPS, the microbial by-product (Wachsmuth et al., 2022). Colonisation with a healthy microbiota restores these signalling pathways and improves glucose homeostasis, whereas recolonisation with a diabetic microbiota fails to achieve similar effects, highlighting the role of microbial composition in neural and metabolic regulation (Wachsmuth et al., 2022; Purdel et al., 2023).

3.3 Diet and Glucose Metabolism

3.3.1 Acute Dietary Effects

Short-term dietary interventions can lead to rapid changes in gut microbiota composition, particularly at the species and family level, within 24 to 48 hours, although the overall microbial structure (enterotype) remains relatively stable. These microbial changes can directly influence the host metabolism by modifying SCFA production, intestinal barrier function, and inflammation, which impacts glucose homeostasis (Singh et al., 2017). Diets high in fat or protein might reduce the number of beneficial bacteria, such as *Eubacterium rectale* and *Roseburia*, which can affect butyrate levels and perhaps impair insulin sensitivity (Davide Menafra et al., 2024). Also, time-restricted feeding and circadian-aligned eating patterns have been shown to affect microbial rhythmicity, which may influence postprandial glucose responses (Severino et al., 2024). However, prolonged dietary changes can induce permanent changes in the gut microbiota. On the other hand, habitual diet has a more consistent and long-lasting effect on gut microbiota composition and metabolic regulation (Singh et al., 2017).

3.3.2 Long-Term Dietary Effects

Long-term adherence to high-fibre, plant-based diets is related to increased microbial diversity and abundance of beneficial taxa like *Bifidobacterium*, *Faecalibacterium prausnitzii*, *Lactobacillus*, and *Akkermansia*, which are linked to improved glucose tolerance and insulin sensitivity (Singh et al., 2017). According to cross-sectional and longitudinal research, people who eat a diet high in plant foods have superior metabolic profiles and more resilient microbiota. On the other hand, Western diets, which are high in fat and sugar and low in fibre, can cause metabolic endotoxemia, a condition linked to insulin resistance and T2D (Piccioni et al., 2023). Moreover, studies showed that the presence of specific bacteria, such as *Akkermansia muciniphila*, may predict individual responsiveness to dietary interventions aimed at improving glucose metabolism. Thus, personalised nutrition based on baseline microbiome composition is emerging as a promising strategy for optimising glucose control (Latif et al., 2023).

3.3.3 Probiotics, Prebiotics, and Synbiotics in Glucose Metabolism

The use of probiotics and prebiotics as dietary interventions has unique mechanisms of action; both aim to enhance the abundance and activity of beneficial gut microbes that influence host metabolic pathways (Chandrasekaran et al., 2024). Probiotics, the live microorganisms that have beneficial effects on the host when ingested in sufficient amounts, have complex and numerous effects on the gut microbiota (Guevara et al., 2024). Strains such as *Lactobacillus, Bifidobacterium,* etc., enhance microbial diversity and stability by competing with pathogens, producing antimicrobial compounds, like bacteriocins, and strengthening gut mucosal barrier functions (Zhao et al., 2019). They also contribute to metabolic regulation by fermentation of carbohydrates into SCFAs, including acetate, propionate, and butyrate, that mediate immune function and regulate intestinal hormone release, such as GLP-1, thereby maintaining appetite and influencing downstream regulation of glucose metabolism. They are known to reduce intestinal inflammation and enhance epithelial barrier function, both of which are critical aspects of decreasing both insulin resistance and systemic metabolic impairments commonly seen in T2D. Prebiotics are selectively fermentable dietary substrates, which are primarily non-digestible carbohydrates like inulin, fructooligosaccharides (FOS), and galacto-oligosaccharides (GOS), that stimulate the growth and activity of beneficial gut bacteria (Singh et al., 2017). Their fermentation by microbes such as *Bifidobacterium*, *Ruminococcus*, and *Eubacterium* results in increased production of SCFAs (Zhang et al., 2019). Studies suggest that synbiotics (combinations of probiotics and prebiotics) are a preferred method to enhance metabolic health. The prebiotic portion of the synbiotic supplements provides the probiotics nutrient niche that will lead to optimal colony and function (Patterson et al., 2016). Studies have shown that synbiotic supplementation can reduce fasting glucose and HbA1c levels, enhance insulin sensitivity and lipid profiles, and decrease systemic inflammation, as reflected by changes in C-reactive protein (CRP) and cytokine levels (Kasubuchi et al., 2015).

4 Gut Microbiota-Derived Metabolites and their Role in Diabetes

4.1 Acetate, Butyrate, and Propionate

The balance and levels of SCFAs are linked with the host's physiological state, with alterations observed in metabolic disorders such as T1D and T2D. In T2D, a noticeable decrease in butyrate production has been reported consistently, while acetate and butyrate tend to increase (Liu et al., 2020). Butyrate, produced by Firmicutes, maintains intestinal homeostasis by nourishing colonocytes, enhancing gut barrier integrity, and modulating inflammation (Larabi et al., 2023). Animal studies have given evidence for the therapeutic potential of SCFAs in managing T2D. For instance, long-term oral acetate administration significantly reduced weight, fat accumulation, and lipogenic gene expression while improving glucose tolerance in diabetic OLETF (Otsuka Long-Evans Tokushima Fatty) rats. Similarly, in diabetic KK-A(y) mice, acetate and propionate reduced blood glucose levels, noting their function in enhancing insulin sensitivity and energy balance. Butyrate has been shown to improve insulin sensitivity and glucose metabolism in humans, indicating its potential as a therapeutic means for the treatment of T2D (Doden & Ridlon, 2021). On the other hand, in T1D, a distinct pattern of SCFA dysregulation emerges, characterised by a decline in butyrate-producing bacteria and reduced overall SCFA production, which coincides with a loss of microbial diversity, indicating a link between gut microbiota composition, impaired butyrate production, and autoimmune responses (Doden & Ridlon, 2021). Butyrate's protective role in altering the immune responses and maintaining epithelial integrity is seen in T1D, where gut barrier function and increased intestinal permeability may provoke autoimmunity. Furthermore, reduced SCFA production is also associated with impaired mucus layer thickness and antimicrobial peptide secretion, weakening host defences and further promoting microbial translocation and systemic inflammation (Zhang et al., 2019).

4.2 Secondary Bile Acids

Secondary bile acids (SBA), produced by the gut microbiota through the conversion of primary bile acids (PBA) secreted by the liver, have recently been recognised as key modulators of glucose metabolism and insulin sensitivity. The metabolites, including deoxycholic acid (DCA) and lithocholic acid (LCA), are more hydrophobic and bioactive than their precursors. These metabolites are formed when gut microbiota, particularly those expressing bile salt hydrolase (BSH) and 7α-dehydroxylation enzymes, act on PBAs. This process is carried out by specific bacterial taxa like *Clostridium scindens*, *Peptacetobacter hiranonis*, and *Clostridium hylemonae* (Zhang et al., 2019). The amphipathic nature of SBAs, with their hydrophobic and hydrophilic properties, also allows them to interact with cell membranes, disrupting bacterial membranes and exerting antimicrobial effects. This aids in regulating the gut microbiota by maintaining a balance between beneficial and pathogenic species (Zhang et al., 2019; Calissi et al., 2020). SBAs play multifaceted roles in glucose homeostasis, lipid metabolism, and inflammation. They function as signalling molecules by binding to receptors like the Farnesoid X receptor (FXR) and Takeda G-protein-coupled receptor 5 (TGR5) (Calissi et al., 2020). Activation of FXR receptors by bile acids regulates gluconeogenesis, glycogen-synthesising lipid metabolism in the liver. Activation of TGR5, on the other hand, stimulates GLP-1 secretion from enteroendocrine cells (EECs), which improves insulin secretion and promotes glycaemic control. Moreover, TGR5-mediated signalling in brown adipose tissue can increase thermogenesis, enhancing energy utilisation and metabolic health (Xu et al., 2020).

4.3 Trimethylamine N-Oxide

Gut microbes including bacterial strains such as *Anaerococcus hydrogenalis*, *Clostridium* spp., *Edwardsiella tarda*, *Escherichia fergusonii*, and others produce trimethylamine (TMA) from choline, carnitine, and betaine, synthesised in the liver via flavin monooxygenase 3 (FOMO3) and excreted through urine. Trimethylamine N-oxide (TMAO) has emerged as a contributing factor for several disorders like metabolic and cardiovascular diseases, including diabetes, by stimulating inflammation, insulin resistance, and metabolic dysfunction. TMA is absorbed and oxidised to TMAO in the liver by flavin monooxygenase (FMO3). While most TMAO is excreted (95% via urine), circulating levels remain elevated in patients with diabetes, highlighting its potential as a biomarker for these conditions and a target for therapeutic strategies (Guo et al., 2023; Romano et al., 2015). Elevated plasma TMAO levels are strongly associated with insulin resistance, puffiness, and oxidative stress, potential contributors to the aetiology of diabetes. Studies suggest that TMAO intensifies vascular dysfunction by promoting endothelial inflammation and lipid deposition, thereby increasing the risk of diabetes-associated cardiovascular complications. Besides, TMAO influences glucose metabolism by impairing mitochondrial function and promoting oxidative stress, which disrupts insulin signalling pathways (Subramaniam & Fletcher, 2017). Recent research studies have also shown that TMAO is linked with chronic low-grade inflammation, a key characteristic feature of T2D, by activating inflammatory markers like interleukin-6 (IL-6) and tumour necrosis factor-alpha (TNF-α). Additionally, TMAO has been linked to altering the gut barrier integrity, which could worsen systemic inflammation and metabolic endotoxemia (Li et al., 2018). Dietary treatments, such as reduced intake of TMAO precursors and using prebiotics to modulate gut microbial composition, have shown promise in lowering TMAO's detrimental effects and improving metabolic outcomes. As a metabolite, TMAO provides valuable insights into treatment approaches for managing diabetes and its complications, highlighting the complex relationship between nutrition, microbial metabolism, and host metabolic health (Brunt et al., 2020).

5 Therapeutic Implications of Targeting Gut Microbiota in Diabetes

5.1 Probiotics

Probiotics are viable microorganisms with health benefits and have shown notable improvements in glycaemic control and insulin sensitivity. The predominant strains are *Bifidobacterium bifidum*, *Lactobacillus acidophilus*, and *Lactobacillus casei* (Ansari et al., 2023), which are particularly effective in producing metabolites of SCFA that interact with G-protein-coupled receptors (e.g. GPR41 and GPR43), reduce systemic inflammation, stimulate GLP-1 release, and enhance insulin sensitivity. These strains also alter immune responses by reducing proinflammatory cytokines through Toll-like receptor pathways and inhibiting nuclear factor kappa B (NF-κB) signalling, thereby reducing the inflammatory response associated with insulin resistance (Markowiak-Kopeć & Śliżewska, 2020). Probiotics have been shown to lower serum CRP levels and improve cardiometabolic parameters in patients with diabetes. Their ability to prevent gut dysbiosis and preserve barrier function underscores their importance in diabetes therapy. Furthermore, dietary fibres have been shown to shift the microbiota metabolism from producing harmful metabolites to synthesising beneficial compounds like SCFAs, linking fibre intake directly to metabolic improvements in patients with T2D (Plovier et al., 2016; Venkataraman et al., 2016).

5.2 Prebiotics

Prebiotics, including fermentable dietary fibres and resistant starches, play a pivotal role by selectively nourishing beneficial gut microbes such as *Bifidobacterium adolescentis* and *Bifidobacterium adolescents* (Camilleri, 2019) These microorganisms produce SCFA metabolites that support metabolic health. Clinical studies have shown that prebiotic supplementation can reduce HbA1c levels, improve fasting glucose levels, and enhance insulin sensitivity as measured by the homeostasis model assessment of insulin resistance (HOMA-IR), particularly with long-term use. In addition, prebiotics help prevent gut dysbiosis and strengthen mucosal barrier function, highlighting their importance in diabetes management (Venkataraman et al., 2016).

5.3 Synbiotics

Synbiotics, the combination of probiotics and prebiotics, offer a synergistic approach by enriching beneficial gut microbes and optimising their activity, leading to improved glycaemic control and overall gut health. Supplementing the diet with synbiotics may help maintain glucose homeostasis and enhance lipid metabolism in patients with type 2 diabetes (T2D). Moreover, synbiotic therapy has been associated with anti-inflammatory effects and reductions in body weight (Ferrarese et al., 2018). For example, a randomised trial demonstrated that synbiotic supplementation significantly improved fasting glucose levels, insulin resistance, and inflammatory markers such as CRP and TNF-α while also enhancing antioxidant capacity. These synergistic effects highlight the therapeutic potential of gut-targeted interventions in the management of metabolic disorders (Ferrarese et al., 2018).

5.4 Fecal Microbiota Transplant (FMT)

Fecal microbiota transplantation (FMT) is the treatment that restores the natural balance of gut microbiota by transferring stool from a healthy donor with normal gut microbiota into a patient with microbial dysbiosis. Studies indicate that FMT can boost insulin sensitivity and reduce systemic inflammation in diabetes by rebalancing dysbiotic microbiota. FMT presumably works by increasing microbial diversity, promoting beneficial bacteria, and reducing the number of detrimental microbes. This can help improve gut barrier function, reduce inflammation, and modulate immune responses, making this a possible strategy for restoring gut health and ultimately preventing disease progression (Valdes et al., 2018).

5.5 Diet and Exercise

Diet and exercise majorly play a pivotal role in modulating the gut microbiota and improving metabolic health, with studies showing that dietary changes explain 57% of microbiota variations compared to 12% of genetic mutations (Craciun et al., 2022). A proper diet is essential for sustaining a healthy gut microbiome, supporting its role in digestion, immunity, and overall metabolic health (Table 1). Diets particularly focus on high-fibre foods rich in fruits, vegetables, and whole grains to promote microbial diversity and increase SCFA production, enhance insulin sensitivity, and prevent mucus layer degradation and microbial encroachment linked to the Western diet. These diets increase the beneficial Bacteroidetes and reduce harmful Firmicutes and Enterobacteriaceae. Similarly, protein sources impact the gut diversity, where plant proteins boost *Bifidobacterium and Lactobacillus*, whereas animal proteins increase *Bacteroides* and other potentially harmful bacteria. Mediterranean diet improve gut microbiota, enhancing insulin sensitivity and glycaemic control. Interventions such as intermittent fasting promote beneficial bacteria like *Akkermansia muciniphila*, though effects are often transient. However, modern dietary factors like artificial sweeteners may disrupt gut balance, including glucose intolerance (Bressa et al., 2017). Regular physical exercise indirectly modulates gut microbiota by influencing gut physiology and morphology. Low-intensity exercise reduces intestinal transit time, while prolonged activity can alter gut permeability. Animal studies have demonstrated that exercise can restore gut microbial balance, increase SCFA concentrations, and reduce the inflammatory state associated with a high diet, making it an essential component in gut-microbiota-targeted

Table 1 Dietary interventions and their effects on gut microbiota in diabetes

Dietary intervention	Key components	Effects on gut microbiota	Impact on diabetes	Ref
High-fibre diet	Whole grains, fruits, vegetables, legumes	Increases SCFA production; enhances *Bifidobacterium* and *Lactobacillus* abundance; reduces systemic inflammation	Improves glycaemic control; reduces insulin resistance	Bressa et al. (2017)
Mediterranean diet	Fruits, vegetables, whole grains, olive oil, fish	Increases diversity of gut microbiota; enhances SCFA production	Reduces HbA1c levels and oxidative stress; improves metabolic health	Bressa et al. (2017)
Low-carbohydrate diet	Reduced carbohydrates, high protein, healthy fats	Reduces Firmicutes/ Bacteroidetes ratio; alters gut microbial composition	Promotes weight loss; improves glucose levels and insulin sensitivity	Saha et al. (2024)
Probiotic supplementation	*Lactobacillus*, *Bifidobacterium* strains	Increases beneficial bacteria (e.g. *Lactobacillus*); reduces gut dysbiosis	Enhances insulin sensitivity; lowers blood glucose and HbA1c levels	Karakan (2020)
Prebiotic diet	Inulin, fructooligosaccharides (FOS), galactooligosaccharides (GOS)	Stimulates growth of *Bifidobacterium* and SCFA producers	Reduces fasting glucose; improves lipid profile	Karakan (2020)
Ketogenic diet	Very low carbohydrates, high fat, moderate protein	Decreases microbial diversity; alters microbiome toward Proteobacteria	Improves blood glucose control short term; potential adverse effects long term	Monda et al. (2017)
Polyphenol-rich diet	Green tea, berries, dark chocolate, red wine	Increases SCFA-producing bacteria; enhances *Bifidobacterium* and *Akkermansia*	Reduces oxidative stress and inflammation; improves glycaemic control	Li et al. (2024)

(continued)

Table 1 (continued)

Dietary intervention	Key components	Effects on gut microbiota	Impact on diabetes	Ref
Omega-3 fatty acid supplementation	Fish oil, flaxseed, walnuts	Enhances *Akkermansia muciniphila* levels; reduces inflammation-associated microbes	Improves insulin sensitivity; reduces chronic inflammation	Ang et al. (2020)
Caloric restriction	Reduced energy intake	Promotes microbial diversity; increases SCFA-producing bacteria	Improves glycaemic control and insulin sensitivity; reduces diabetes complications	Yang et al. (2020)

Overview of dietary interventions, their impact on gut microbiota composition and function, and the resulting effects on diabetes parameters such as glycaemic control, insulin sensitivity, and inflammation

strategies. It can also counteract the effects of a high-fat diet by improving the Bacteroidetes/Firmicutes ratio. While human study evidence remains limited, these findings highlight the combined potential of diet and exercise to positively impact gut microbiota and improve metabolic health in diabetes management (Saha et al., 2024).

5.6 Personalised Nutrition

Personalised nutrition and medicine utilise individual differences, such as gut microbiota composition, to optimise therapeutic outcomes. Research by (Zeevi et al., 2015) demonstrated that machine learning algorithms integrating clinical and microbiota data could reliably predict individual glucose responses. In clinical trials, personalised dietary interventions successfully normalised blood glucose levels. Similarly, studies examining dietary responses, such as glycaemic variability to different types of bread, highlight the predictive value of microbiome profiling in tailoring effective therapies. However, further research is needed to better understand the variability, sustainability, and long-term benefits of such individualised approaches (Zivkovic et al., 2011; Tanca et al., 2018). Given this, gut microbiota modulation shows strong potential in the control and prevention of both T1D and T2D. Microbiota-targeted strategies help restore microbial balance, strengthen gut barrier integrity, and regulate immune responses. Clinical and experimental studies have demonstrated their ability to lower fasting blood glucose and HbA1c levels, reduce insulin resistance, and improve insulin sensitivity and inflammatory markers (Korem et al., 2017). The overall therapeutic application of gut microbiota in diabetes is summarised in Fig. 4.

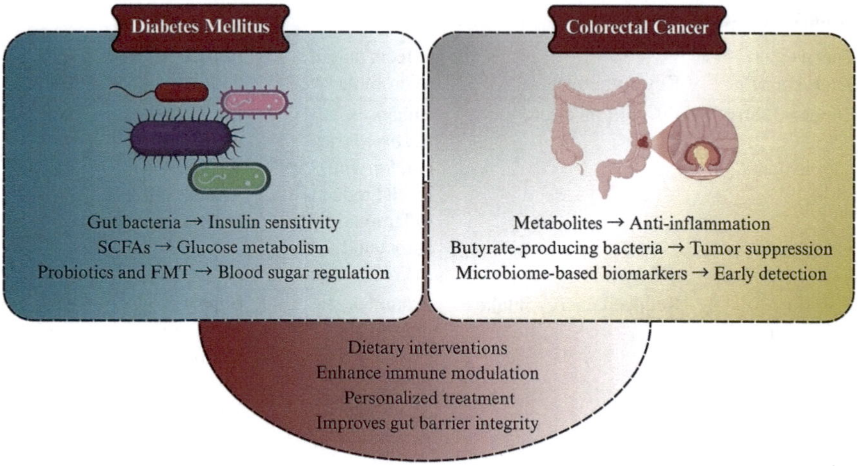

Fig. 4 Clinical applications of gut microbiota in diabetes and colorectal cancer, emphasising their therapeutic and diagnostic potential

6 Gut Microbiota as a Link Between Diabetes Mellitus and Colorectal Cancer

The gut microbiota has emerged not only as a key regulator of metabolic diseases such as diabetes mellitus but also as an important player in cancer development, particularly CRC (Song & Chan, 2019). Accumulating evidence suggests that dysbiosis serves as a shared pathological link between diabetes and CRC, largely through mechanisms involving chronic inflammation, altered gut permeability, immune dysregulation, and metabolic endotoxemia (Zhao et al., 2023). Gut microbiota is a critical common nexus linking diabetes mellitus, particularly T2D, with CRC through gut microbial dysbiosis-mediated regulation of chronic inflammation, metabolic derangements, and immune disturbances. In T2D, dysbiosis is defined as the loss of commensal butyrate-producing bacteria with a gain of pathogenic taxa that compromises intestinal barrier function and drives a proinflammatory environment. This dysregulation results in overexpression of proinflammatory cytokines like interleukin-1β (IL-1β) and enzymes like NADPH oxidase 4 (NOX4), promoting oxidative stress through reactive oxygen species (ROS) that induce damage in colonic epithelial cells and promote carcinogenesis. Experimental models involving diabetic mice have reported that transplantation of fecal microbiota from mice with diabetic or CRC into normal mice enhances colon polyp development, validating the active contribution of diabetes-related microbial changes to CRC development (Noureldein et al., 2022). Further, CRC patients have diminished microbial diversity and increased pro-carcinogenic bacteria like *Fusobacterium nucleatum* and *Bacteroides*, which facilitate tumorigenesis through the promotion of inflammation, DNA damage, and immune evasion (Gao et al., 2017; Russ et al., 2024). Gut microbiota-derived metabolites such as secondary bile acids, TMAO, SCFAs, and other compounds such as hydrogen sulphide and N-nitroso also perform vital functions by stimulating carcinogenic signalling pathways (e.g. Wnt/β-catenin, EGFR-ERK1/2) and causing DNA damage and hence directly connecting metabolic dysregulation in diabetes to the pathogenesis of CRC (Zhang et al., 2021). Chronic low-grade inflammation, a characteristic common to obesity, diabetes, and CRC, is increased by gut dysbiosis, leading to disruption of immune homeostasis and a tumorigenesis-supporting microenvironment (Rumyantsev et al., 2024; Gutiérrez-Salmerón et al., 2021). Therapeutic strategies aimed at the gut microbiota, including probiotics that reconstitute butyrate-producing bacteria and inhibit inflammatory mediators, have been found to decrease CRC risk and reverse diabetes-associated gastrointestinal complications (Zhao et al., 2023; Sadagopan et al., 2023).

7 Challenges of Microbiota-Targeted Therapy in Diabetes

The gut microbiome holds great promise in managing diabetes. Although there has been a lot of research on diabetes and gut microbiota, there are notable limitations that must be addressed. One of the main challenges is the extensive variation of gut bacteria between individuals, determined by factors such as genetics, diet, lifestyle, environment, and medication usage, so it is hard to make universal therapeutic approaches (Schupack et al., 2022). Multiple mechanisms that connect microbes in the gut to glucose metabolism and insulin sensitivity remain complex (Silva et al., 2020). There is still uncertainty regarding which bacterial strains are most beneficial, what the optimal doses are, and the appropriate duration of treatment (Li et al., 2020). Most studies until now have observed short-term benefits, which involve small sample sizes, and the long-term consequences of modifying the microbiota are yet to be understood (Baldi et al., 2021). Another limitation is the use of animals for the study. Germ-free animals, which are born and raised without exposure to any bacteria, are predominantly used in experiments and are introduced to specific microbes during the research process. Furthermore, individuals responding to treatments including probiotics, prebiotics, and faecal microbiota transplantation vary widely, making it more difficult to develop treatments that are effective for everyone (Rebersek, 2021). Current methods for evaluating and modulating the gut microbiota are still evolving. To fully harness their potential in diabetes management, larger, long-term studies and personalized approaches are needed.

8 Applications of the Gut Microbiome in Clinical Practice for Colorectal Cancer

The gut microbiome is central to the clinical management of CRC, providing applications in screening, prognosis, prediction of treatment, and therapeutic modulation (Fig. 4). As a screening biomarker, microbial taxa like *Fusobacterium nucleatum*, identified from faecal material, are enriched in those with adenomas or CRC, allowing early and noninvasive detection (Cheng et al., 2020). Metabolic and genotoxic metabolites of individual microbes also provide early markers. As predictive and prognostic biomarkers, the gut microbiota can predict patient outcomes, treatment efficacy, and toxicity (Cheng et al., 2020). Microbial genes, metabolites, faecal, tumour tissue, or blood serological markers guide precision CRC therapy. Gut microbiome modulation is being shown to be a potent means of preventing CRC and maximising chemotherapy and immunotherapy efficacy and tolerability (Fong et al., 2020). Strategies involve dietary intervention, probiotics, prebiotics, and synbiotics, which together promote healthy microbial populations, enhance gut barrier function, inhibit inflammation, and inactivate carcinogens. Particularly, FMT is emerging as a new biotherapeutic approach. Through the transfer of faecal material from healthy donors, FMT reestablishes microbial balance and has been clinically effective in the treatment of *Clostridioides difficile* infection and immune-related colitis (Valdes et al., 2018). Although still under investigation for CRC, preclinical studies indicate that FMT can suppress tumorigenesis and increase host resistance. Further, FMT has shown promise in reversing colitis induced by immunotherapy, highlighting its wider utility in cancer treatment. Collectively, these microbiome-directed therapies are novel, nonsurgical, and personalised therapies for the management of CRC and better patient outcomes.

9 Conclusion and Future Perspectives

Gut microbiota is key factor in the regulation of glucose homeostasis and pathophysiology of diabetes mellitus. Dysbiosis not only causes insulin resistance and systemic inflammation but also creates a connection to CRC via metabolic and immunologic abnormality. The common mechanisms between diabetes and CRC emphasize the gut microbiota as a key therapeutic target for both metabolic and oncologic disorders. Novel microbiota-directed approaches, such as probiotics, prebiotics, synbiotics, dietary management, and fecal microbiota transplantation, hold great promise in controlling these interrelated conditions. But future studies need to concentrate on individualised strategies, safety over the long term, and mechanistic understanding to maximise the application of microbiome-based therapies to integrate disease prevention and care. The role of gut microbiota in managing diabetes presents exciting opportunities for new, personalised treatments. Future research should focus on better understanding how each gut bacteria influence glucose levels, insulin resistance, and immunity. Extensive, long-term studies involving human participants are necessary to validate these findings and minimise dependence on animal experiments. Standardising methods for analysing the gut microbiome, such as genetic sequencing and stool processing, will make research findings more consistent. Advanced tools like machine learning could also help to identify specific bacteria linked to diabetes, enabling the design of more targeted therapies. Personalised treatments using probiotics, prebiotics, and faecal microbiota transplants offer significant potential but require rigorous research to determine the safest and most effective approaches. It is important to explore the right combination of bacterial strains, dosages, and treatment durations, along with their long-term effects. Combining these microbiota-based therapies with healthy diets, exercise, and lifestyle changes could provide a holistic approach to diabetes care. This holistic approach or the interplay between gut microbiota and systemic health suggests a possibility of prevention of not only diabetes but also its complications, thereby emphasising the need for a multidisciplinary approach in future research.

Acknowledgements The authors are thankful to Chettinad Academy of Research and Education (CARE) for providing the infrastructural and financial support.

Conflict of Interest None. All authors declare that there are no conflicts of or competing interests.

Authors' Contributions AB and AR conceptualised the chapter. NSS, SN, ASP, and AB were involved in manuscript preparation and pictorial representations. NSS, SN, and ASP designed the images and tables. AB and AR have critically reviewed the draft manuscript and provided feedback on writing and editing. All authors have read and approved the final manuscript.

Funding The authors acknowledge the financial support provided by Chettinad Academy of Research and Education (CARE) to complete the work. NSS acknowledges Chettinad Academy of Research and Education (CARE) for providing the JRF fellowship.

References

Ahola, A. J., Lassenius, M. I., Forsblom, C., Harjutsalo, V., Lehto, M., & Groop, P.-H. (2017). Dietary patterns reflecting healthy food choices are associated with lower serum LPS activity. *Scientific Reports, 7*(1). https://doi.org/10.1038/s41598-017-06885-7

Campbell, J. E., & Drucker, D. J. (2015). Islet α cells and glucagon—critical regulators of energy homeostasis. *Nature Reviews Endocrinology, 11*(6), 329–338. https://doi.org/10.1038/nrendo.2015.51

Ang, Q. Y., Alexander, M., Newman, J. C., Tian, Y., Cai, J., Upadhyay, V., Turnbaugh, J. A., Verdin, E., Hall, K. D., Leibel, R. L., Ravussin, E., Rosenbaum, M., Patterson, A. D., & Turnbaugh, P. J. (2020). Ketogenic diets alter the gut microbiome resulting in decreased intestinal Th17 cells. *Cell, 181*(6). https://doi.org/10.1016/j.cell.2020.04.027

Ansari, F., Neshat, M., Pourjafar, H., Jafari, S. M., Samakkhah, S. A., & Mirzakhani, E. (2023). The role of probiotics and prebiotics in modulating of the gut-brain axis. *Frontiers in Nutrition, 10*. https://doi.org/10.3389/fnut.2023.1173660

Baldi, S., Mundula, T., Nannini, G., & Amedei, A. (2021). Microbiota shaping - the effects of probiotics, prebiotics, and fecal microbiota transplant on cognitive functions: A systematic review. *World Journal of Gastroenterology, 27*(39), 6715–6732. https://doi.org/10.3748/wjg.v27.i39.6715

Banday, M., Sameer, A., & Nissar, S. (2020). Pathophysiology of diabetes: An overview. *Avicenna Journal of Medicine, 10*(4), 174–188. https://doi.org/10.4103/ajm.ajm_53_20

Bielka, W., Przezak, A., & Pawlik, A. (2022). The role of the gut microbiota in the pathogenesis of diabetes. *International Journal of Molecular Sciences, 23*(1), 480. https://doi.org/10.3390/ijms23010480

Breit, S., Kupferberg, A., Rogler, G., & Hasler, G. (2018). Vagus nerve as modulator of the brain–gut axis in psychiatric and inflammatory disorders. *Frontiers in Psychiatry, 9*(44). https://doi.org/10.3389/fpsyt.2018.00044

Bressa, C., Bailén-Andrino, M., Pérez-Santiago, J., González-Soltero, R., Pérez, M., Montalvo-Lominchar, M. G., Maté-Muñoz, J. L., Domínguez, R., Moreno, D., & Larrosa, M. (2017). The role of the gut microbiota in the pathogenesis of diabetes. *PLoS One, 12*(2), e0171352. https://doi.org/10.1371/journal.pone.0171352

Brunt, V. E., LaRocca, T. J., Bazzoni, A. E., Sapinsley, Z. J., Miyamoto-Ditmon, J., Gioscia-Ryan, R. A., Neilson, A. P., Link, C. D., & Seals, D. R. (2020). The gut microbiome–derived metabolite trimethylamine N-oxide modulates neuroinflammation and cognitive function with aging. *GeroScience, 43*(1), 377–394. https://doi.org/10.1007/s11357-020-00257-2

Cai, Y., Liu, Y., Wu, Z., Wang, J., & Zhang, X. (2023). Effects of diet and exercise on circadian rhythm: Role of gut microbiota in immune and metabolic systems. *Nutrients, 15*(12), 2743–2743. https://doi.org/10.3390/nu15122743

Calissi, G., Lam, E. W.-F., & Link, W. (2020). Therapeutic strategies targeting FOXO transcription factors. *Nature Reviews Drug Discovery.* https://doi.org/10.1038/s41573-020-0088-2

Camilleri, M. (2019). Leaky gut: Mechanisms, measurement and clinical implications in humans. *Gut, 68*(8), 1516–1526. https://doi.org/10.1136/gutjnl-2019-318427

Chandrasekaran, P., Weiskirchen, S., & Weiskirchen, R. (2024). Effects of probiotics on gut microbiota: An overview. *International Journal of Molecular Sciences, 25*(11), 6022. https://doi.org/10.3390/ijms25116022

Cheng, Y., Ling, Z., & Li, L. (2020). The intestinal microbiota and colorectal cancer. *Frontiers in Immunology, 11*. https://doi.org/10.3389/fimmu.2020.615056

Chia, C. W., & Egan, J. M. (2019). Incretins in obesity and diabetes. *Annals of the New York Academy of Sciences, 1461*(1), 104–126. https://doi.org/10.1111/nyas.14211

Craciun, C.-I., Neag, M.-A., Catinean, A., Mitre, A.-O., Rusu, A., Bala, C., Roman, G., Buzoianu, A.-D., Muntean, D.-M., & Craciun, A.-E. (2022). The relationships between gut microbiota and diabetes mellitus, and treatments for diabetes mellitus. *Biomedicine, 10*(2), 308. https://doi.org/10.3390/biomedicines10020308

Dash, S., Syed, Y. A., & Khan, M. R. (2022). Understanding the role of the gut microbiome in brain development and its association with neurodevelopmental psychiatric disorders. *Frontiers in Cell and Developmental Biology, 10*. https://doi.org/10.3389/fcell.2022.880544

Davide Menafra, Mattia Proganò, Tecce, N., Pivonello, R., & Colao, A. (2024). Diet and gut microbiome: Impact of each factor and mutual interactions on prevention and treatment of type 2, type 1, and gestational diabetes. *Human Nutrition & Metabolism*, 200286. https://doi.org/10.1016/j.hnm.2024.200286

Doden, H. L., & Ridlon, J. M. (2021). Microbial Hydroxysteroid dehydrogenases: From alpha to omega. *Microorganisms, 9*(3), 469–469. https://doi.org/10.3390/microorganisms9030469

El-Zayat, S. R., Sibaii, H., & Mannaa, F. A. (2019). Toll-like receptors activation, signaling, and targeting: An overview. *Bulletin of the National Research Centre, 43*(1). https://doi.org/10.1186/s42269-019-0227-2

Ferrarese, R., Ceresola, E. R., Preti, A., & Canducci, F. (2018). Probiotics, prebiotics and synbiotics for weight loss and metabolic syndrome in the microbiome era. *European Review for Medical and Pharmacological Sciences, 22*(21), 7588–7605. https://doi.org/10.26355/eurrev_201811_16301

Frolova, M. S., Suvorova, I. A., Iablokov, S. N., Petrov, S. N., & Rodionov, D. A. (2022). Genomic reconstruction of short-chain fatty acid production by the human gut microbiota. *Frontiers in Molecular Biosciences, 9*. https://doi.org/10.3389/fmolb.2022.949563

Fong, W., Li, Q., & Yu, J. (2020). Gut microbiota modulation: A novel strategy for prevention and treatment of colorectal cancer. *Oncogene, 39*(26), 4925–4943. https://doi.org/10.1038/s41388-020-1341-1

Gao, R., Gao, Z., Huang, L., & Qin, H. (2017). Gut microbiota and colorectal cancer. *European Journal of Clinical Microbiology & Infectious Diseases, 36*(5), 757–769. https://doi.org/10.1007/s10096-016-2881-8

Guevara, D. M., Cañas, S. V., Palacios, I., Gómez, A., Estrada, M., Gallego, J., & Liscano, Y. (2024). Effectiveness of probiotics, prebiotics, and synbiotics in managing insulin resistance and hormonal imbalance in women with polycystic ovary syndrome (PCOS): A systematic review of randomized clinical trials. *Nutrients, 16*(22), 3916–3916. https://doi.org/10.3390/nu16223916

Guo, H., Wu, H., & Li, Z. (2023). The pathogenesis of diabetes. *International Journal of Molecular Sciences, 24*(8), 6978. https://doi.org/10.3390/ijms24086978

Gutiérrez-Salmerón, M., Lucena, S. R. R., Chocarro-Calvo, A., Garcia-Martinez, J. M., Martín Orozco, R. M., & García-Jiménez, C. (2021). Remodelling of colorectal cancer cell signaling by microbiota and immunity in diabetes. *Endocrine-Related Cancer.* https://doi.org/10.1530/erc-20-0315

He, J., Zhang, P., Shen, L., Niu, L., Tan, Y., Chen, L., Zhao, Y., Bai, L., Hao, X., Li, X., Zhang, S., & Zhu, L. (2020). Short-chain fatty acids and their association with signalling pathways in inflammation, glucose and lipid metabolism. *International Journal of Molecular Sciences, 21*(17), 6356. https://doi.org/10.3390/ijms21176356

Ho, J. T., Chan, G. C., & Li, J. C. (2015). Systemic effects of gut microbiota and its relationship with disease and modulation. *BMC Immunology, 16*(1). https://doi.org/10.1186/s12865-015-0083-2

Hossain, M. J., Al-Mamun, M., & Islam, M. R. (2024). Diabetes mellitus, the fastest growing global public health concern: Early detection should be focused. *Health Science Reports, 7*(3), e2004. https://doi.org/10.1002/hsr2.2004

Johanns, M., Hue, L., & Rider, M. H. (2023). AMPK inhibits liver gluconeogenesis: Fact or fiction? *Biochemical Journal, 480*(1), 105–125. https://doi.org/10.1042/bcj20220582

Karakan, T. (2020). Intermittent fasting and gut microbiota. *The Turkish Journal of Gastroenterology, 30*(12), 1008–1008. https://doi.org/10.5152/tjg.2019.101219

Kasubuchi, M., Hasegawa, S., Hiramatsu, T., Ichimura, A., & Kimura, I. (2015). Dietary gut microbial metabolites, short-chain fatty acids, and host metabolic regulation. *Nutrients, 7*(4), 2839–2849. https://doi.org/10.3390/nu7042839

Korem, T., Zeevi, D., Zmora, N., Weissbrod, O., Bar, N., Lotan-Pompan, M., Avnit-Sagi, T., Kosower, N., Malka, G., Rein, M., Suez, J., Goldberg, B. Z., Weinberger, A., Levy, A. A., Elinav, E., & Segal, E. (2017). Bread affects clinical parameters and induces gut microbiome-associated personal glycemic responses. *Cell Metabolism, 25*(6), 1243–1253.e5. https://doi.org/10.1016/j.cmet.2017.05.002

Kumar, S. B., Arnipalli, S. R., & Ziouzenkova, O. (2020). Antibiotics in food chain: The consequences for antibiotic resistance. *Antibiotics, 9*(10), 688. https://doi.org/10.3390/antibiotics9100688

Lange, O., Proczko-Stepaniak, M., & Mika, A. (2023). Short-chain fatty acids—A product of the microbiome and its participation in two-way communication on the microbiome-host mammal line. *Current Obesity Reports, 12*(2), 108–126. https://doi.org/10.1007/s13679-023-00503-6

Larabi, A. B., Masson, H. L. P., & Bäumler, A. J. (2023). Bile acids as modulators of gut microbiota composition and function. *Gut Microbes, 15*(1). https://doi.org/10.1080/19490976.2023.2172671

Latif, A., Shehzad, A., Niazi, S., Zahid, A., Ashraf, W., Iqbal, M. W., Rehman, A., Riaz, T., Aadil, R. M., Khan, I., Özogul, F., Rocha, J. M., Esatbeyoglu, T., & Korma, S. A. (2023). Probiotics: Mechanism of action, health benefits and their application in food industries. *Frontiers in Microbiology, 14*(14). https://doi.org/10.3389/fmicb.2023.1216674

Leeming, E. R., Johnson, A. J., Spector, T. D., & Le Roy, C. I. (2019). Effect of diet on the gut microbiota: Rethinking intervention duration. *Nutrients, 11*(12), 2862. https://doi.org/10.3390/nu11122862

Li, D., Ke, Y., Zhan, R., Liu, C., Zhao, M., Zeng, A., Shi, X., Ji, L., Cheng, S., Pan, B., Zheng, L., & Hong, H. (2018). Trimethylamine-N-oxide promotes brain aging and cognitive impairment in mice. *Aging Cell, 17*(4), e12768. https://doi.org/10.1111/acel.12768

Li, F., McClain, C. J., & Feng, W. (2019). Microbiome dysbiosis and alcoholic liver disease. *Liver Research, 3*(3–4), 218–226. https://doi.org/10.1016/j.livres.2019.09.001

Li, W.-Z., Stirling, K., Yang, J.-J., & Zhang, L. (2020). Gut microbiota and diabetes: From correlation to causality and mechanism. *World Journal of Diabetes, 11*(7), 293–308. https://doi.org/10.4239/wjd.v11.i7.293

Li, L., Li, R., Tian, Q., Luo, Y., Li, R., Lin, X., Ou, Y., Guo, T., Chen, X., Pan, A., Manson, J. E., & Liu, G. (2024). Effects of healthy low-carbohydrate diet and time-restricted eating on weight and gut microbiome in adults with overweight or obesity: Feeding RCT. *Cell Reports Medicine*, 101801. https://doi.org/10.1016/j.xcrm.2024.101801

Liu, J.-L., Segovia, I., Yuan, X.-L., & Gao, Z. (2020). Controversial roles of gut microbiota-derived short-chain fatty acids (SCFAs) on pancreatic β-cell growth and insulin secretion. *International Journal of Molecular Sciences, 21*(3), 910. https://doi.org/10.3390/ijms21030910

Ma, Q., Li, Y., Li, P., Wang, M., Wang, J., Tang, Z., Wang, T., Luo, L., Wang, C., Wang, T., & Zhao, B. (2019). Research progress in the relationship between type 2 diabetes mellitus and intestinal flora. *Biomedicine & Pharmacotherapy, 117*, 109138. https://doi.org/10.1016/j.biopha.2019.109138

Markowiak-Kopeć, P., & Śliżewska, K. (2020). The effect of probiotics on the production of short-chain fatty acids by human intestinal microbiome. *Nutrients, 12*(4), 1107. https://doi.org/10.3390/nu12041107

Martín, R., Bermúdez-Humarán, L. G., & Langella, P. (2018). Searching for the bacterial effector: The example of the multi-skilled commensal bacterium Faecalibacterium prausnitzii. *Frontiers in Microbiology, 9*. https://doi.org/10.3389/fmicb.2018.00346

McVey Neufeld, K. A., Mao, Y. K., Bienenstock, J., Foster, J. A., & Kunze, W. A. (2012). The microbiome is essential for normal gut intrinsic primary afferent neuron excitability in the mouse. *Neurogastroenterology & Motility, 25*(2), 183–e88. https://doi.org/10.1111/nmo.12049

McVey Neufeld, K. A., Perez-Burgos, A., Mao, Y. K., Bienenstock, J., & Kunze, W. A. (2015). The gut microbiome restores intrinsic and extrinsic nerve function in germ-free mice accompanied by changes in calbindin. *Neurogastroenterology & Motility, 27*(5), 627–636. https://doi.org/10.1111/nmo.12534

Milionis, C., Ilias, I., Venaki, E., & Koukkou, E. (2023). Glucose homeostasis, Diabetes mellitus, and gender-affirming treatment. *Biomedicine, 11*(3), 670. https://doi.org/10.3390/biomedicines11030670

Mitoiu, B. I., Nartea, R., & Miclaus, R. S. (2024). Impact of resistance and endurance training on ghrelin and plasma leptin levels in overweight and obese subjects. *International Journal of Molecular Sciences, 25*(15), 8067–8067. https://doi.org/10.3390/ijms25158067

Monda, V., Villano, I., Messina, A., Valenzano, A., Esposito, T., Moscatelli, F., Viggiano, A., Cibelli, G., Chieffi, S., Monda, M., & Messina, G. (2017). Exercise modifies the gut microbiota with positive health effects. *Oxidative Medicine and Cellular Longevity, 2017*, 1–8. https://doi.org/10.1155/2017/3831972

Nandwana, V., Nandwana, N. K., Das, Y., Saito, M., Panda, T., Das, S., Almaguel, F., Hosmane, N. S., & Das, B. C. (2022). The role of microbiome in brain development and neurodegenerative diseases. *Molecules, 27*(11), 3402. https://doi.org/10.3390/molecules27113402

Nauck, M. A., & Meier, J. J. (2018). Incretin hormones: Their role in health and disease. *Diabetes, Obesity & Metabolism, 20 Suppl 1*(S1), 5–21. https://doi.org/10.1111/dom.13129

Noureldein, M., Nawfal, R., Bitar, S., Maxwell, S. S., Khurana, I., Kassouf, H. K., Khuri, F. R., El-Osta, A., & Eid, A. A. (2022). Intestinal microbiota regulates diabetes and cancer progression by IL-1β and NOX4 dependent signaling cascades. *Cellular and Molecular Life Sciences, 79*(9). https://doi.org/10.1007/s00018-022-04485-x

Patloka, O., Komprda, T., & Franke, G. (2024). Review of the relationships between human gut microbiome, diet, and obesity. *Nutrients, 16*(23), 3996–3996. https://doi.org/10.3390/nu16233996

Patterson, E., Ryan, P. M., Cryan, J. F., Dinan, T. G., Ross, R. P., Fitzgerald, G. F., & Stanton, C. (2016). Gut microbiota, obesity and diabetes. *Postgraduate Medical Journal, 92*(1087), 286–300. https://doi.org/10.1136/postgradmedj-2015-133285

Piccioni, A., Covino, M., Candelli, M., Ojetti, V., Capacci, A., Gasbarrini, A., Franceschi, F., & Merra, G. (2023). How do diet patterns, single foods, prebiotics and probiotics impact gut microbiota? *Microbiology Research, 14*(1), 390–408. https://doi.org/10.3390/microbiolres14010030

Plovier, H., Everard, A., Druart, C., Depommier, C., Van Hul, M., Geurts, L., Chilloux, J., Ottman, N., Duparc, T., Lichtenstein, L., Myridakis, A., Delzenne, N. M., Klievink, J., Bhattacharjee, A., van der Ark, K. C. H., Aalvink, S., Martinez, L. O., Dumas, M.-E., Maiter, D., & Loumaye, A. (2016). A purified membrane protein from Akkermansia muciniphila or the pasteurized bacterium improves metabolism in obese and diabetic mice. *Nature Medicine, 23*(1), 107–113. https://doi.org/10.1038/nm.4236

Purdel, C., Margină, D., Adam-Dima, I., & Ungurianu, A. (2023). The beneficial effects of dietary interventions on gut microbiota-An up-to-date critical review and future perspectives. *Nutrients, 15*(23), 5005. https://doi.org/10.3390/nu15235005

Rajan, A., Karpagavel, L., Vidya, S., Sheena, K. S., Harilal, M. D., Deepthi, S., et al. (2024). Correlation of inflammatory markers and NFATC4 gene expression among subjects with prediabetes. *Journal of Cardiovascular and Thoracic Research, 16*(4), 264–274. Rahman, S. (2021). Role of insulin in health and disease: An update. *International Journal of Molecular Sciences, 22*(12), 6403. https://doi.org/10.3390/ijms22126403.

Ramadevi, S., & Meenakshi, S. (2023). Communication with gut microbiota: An emerging strategy to predict and prevent cancer. In R. Sobti, R. C. Kuhad, R. Lal, & P. Rishi (Eds.), *Role of microbes in sustainable development*. Springer. https://doi.org/10.1007/978-981-99-3126-2_21

Rebersek, M. (2021). Gut microbiome and its role in colorectal cancer. *BMC Cancer, 21*(1). https://doi.org/10.1186/s12885-021-09054-2

Rinninella, E., Raoul, P., Cintoni, M., Franceschi, F., Miggiano, G., Gasbarrini, A., & Mele, M. (2019). What is the healthy gut microbiota composition? A changing ecosystem across age, environment, diet, and diseases. *Microorganisms, 7*(1), 14. https://doi.org/10.3390/microorganisms7010014

Romano, K. A., Vivas, E. I., Amador-Noguez, D., & Rey, F. E. (2015). Intestinal microbiota composition modulates choline bioavailability from diet and accumulation of the proatherogenic metabolite trimethylamine-N-oxide. *MBio, 6*(2). https://doi.org/10.1128/mbio.02481-14

Rumyantsev, K. A., Polyakova, V. V., Sorokina, I. V., Feoktistova, P. S., Khatkov, I. E., Bodunova, N. A., & Zhukova, L. G. (2024). The gut microbiota impacts gastrointestinal cancers through obesity, diabetes, and chronic inflammation. *Life (Basel, Switzerland), 14*(10), 1219. https://doi.org/10.3390/life14101219

Russ, C. A., Zertalis, N. A., & Nanton, V. (2024). Gut bacterial microbiome profiles associated with colorectal cancer risk: A narrative review and meta-analysis. *EMJ Gastroenterology*. 10.33590/emjgastroenterol/ohyp9967.

Sadagopan, A., Mahmoud, A., Begg, M., Tarhuni, M., Fotso, M., Gonzalez, N. A., Sanivarapu, R. R., Osman, U., Latha Kumar, A., & Mohammed, L. (2023). Understanding the role of the gut microbiome in diabetes and therapeutics targeting leaky gut: A systematic review. *Cureus, 15*(7), e41559. https://doi.org/10.7759/cureus.41559

Saeedi, P., Petersohn, I., Salpea, P., Malanda, B., Karuranga, S., Unwin, N., Colagiuri, S., Guariguata, L., Motala, A. A., Ogurtsova, K., Shaw, J. E., Bright, D., Williams, R., & IDF Diabetes Atlas Committee. (2019). Global and regional diabetes prevalence estimates for 2019 and projections for 2030 and 2045: Results from the International Diabetes Federation Diabetes Atlas, 9th edition. *Diabetes Research and Clinical Practice, 157*, 107843. https://doi.org/10.1016/j.diabres.2019.107843

Saha, B., T, R. A., Subhamay Adhikary, Banerjee, A., Arun Kumar Radhakrishnan, Duttaroy, A. K., & Pathak, S. (2024). Exploring the relationship between diet, lifestyle and gut microbiome in colorectal cancer development: A recent update. *Nutrition and Cancer, 76*(9), 1–26. https://doi.org/10.1080/01635581.2024.2367266

Sbihi, H., Boutin, R. C. T., Cutler, C., Suen, M., Finlay, B. B., & Turvey, S. E. (2019). Thinking bigger: How early-life environmental exposures shape the gut microbiome and influence the development of asthma and allergic disease. *Allergy, 74*(11), 2103–2115. https://doi.org/10.1111/all.13812

Schupack, D. A., Mars, R. A. T., Voelker, D. H., Abeykoon, J. P., & Kashyap, P. C. (2022). The promise of the gut microbiome as part of individualized treatment strategies. *Nature Reviews Gastroenterology & Hepatology, 19*(1), 7–25. https://doi.org/10.1038/s41575-021-00499-1

Senghor, B., Sokhna, C., Ruimy, R., & Lagier, J. C. (2018). Gut microbiota diversity according to dietary habits and geographical provenance. *Human Microbiome Journal, 7-8*, 1–9. https://doi.org/10.1016/j.humic.2018.01.001

Severino, A., Ege Tohumcu, Tamai, L., Dargenio, P., Porcari, S., Rondinella, D., Venturini, I., Maida, M., Gasbarrini, A., Cammarota, G., & Ianiro, G. (2024). The microbiome-driven impact of Western diet in the development of noncommunicable chronic disorders. *Best Practice & Research Clinical Gastroenterology*, 101923. https://doi.org/10.1016/j.bpg.2024.101923

Sharlize Pedroza Matute, & Sasitaran Iyavoo. (2023). Exploring the gut microbiota: Lifestyle choices, disease associations, and personal genomics. *Frontiers in Nutrition, 10*. https://doi.org/10.3389/fnut.2023.1225120

Shreiner, A. B., Kao, J. Y., & Young, V. B. (2015). The gut microbiome in health and in disease. *Current Opinion in Gastroenterology, 31*(1), 69–75. https://doi.org/10.1097/mog.0000000000000139

Silva, D. R., Sardi, J. D. C. O., de Souza Pitangui, N., Roque, S. M., da Silva, A. C. B., & Rosalen, P. L. (2020). Probiotics as an alternative antimicrobial therapy: Current reality and future directions. *Journal of Functional Foods, 73*, 104080. https://doi.org/10.1016/j.jff.2020.104080

Singh, R. K., Chang, H.-W., Yan, D., Lee, K. M., Ucmak, D., Wong, K., Abrouk, M., Farahnik, B., Nakamura, M., Zhu, T. H., Bhutani, T., & Liao, W. (2017). Influence of diet on the gut microbiome and implications for human health. *Journal of Translational Medicine, 15*(1). https://doi.org/10.1186/s12967-017-1175-y

Singh, S., Sharma, P., Pal, N., Kumawat, M., Shubham, S., Sarma, D. K., Tiwari, R. R., Kumar, M., & Nagpal, R. (2022). Impact of environmental pollutants on gut microbiome and mental health via the gut–brain axis. *Microorganisms, 10*(7), 1457. https://doi.org/10.3390/microorganisms10071457

Song, M., & Chan, A. T. (2019). Environmental factors, gut microbiota, and colorectal cancer prevention. *Clinical Gastroenterology and Hepatology: The Official Clinical Practice Journal of the American Gastroenterological Association, 17*(2), 275–289. https://doi.org/10.1016/j.cgh.2018.07.012

Subramaniam, S., & Fletcher, C. (2017). Trimethylamine N-oxide: Breathe new life. *British Journal of Pharmacology, 175*(8), 1344–1353. https://doi.org/10.1111/bph.13959

Suganya, K., & Koo, B.-S. (2020). Gut–brain axis: role of gut microbiota on neurological disorders and how probiotics/prebiotics beneficially modulate microbial and immune pathways to improve brain functions. *International Journal of Molecular Sciences, 21*(20), 7551. https://doi.org/10.3390/ijms21207551

Tanca, A., Abbondio, M., Palomba, A., Fraumene, C., Marongiu, F., Serra, M., Pagnozzi, D., Laconi, E., & Uzzau, S. (2018). Caloric restriction promotes functional changes involving short-chain fatty acid biosynthesis in the rat gut microbiota. *Scientific Reports, 8*(1). https://doi.org/10.1038/s41598-018-33100-y

Thursby, E., & Juge, N. (2017). Introduction to the human gut microbiota. *Biochemical Journal, 474*(11), 1823–1836. https://doi.org/10.1042/bcj20160510

Valdes, A. M., Walter, J., Segal, E., & Spector, T. D. (2018). Role of the gut microbiota in nutrition and health. *BMJ (Clinical research ed.), 361*(361), k2179. https://doi.org/10.1136/bmj.k2179

Vallianou, N. G., Stratigou, T., & Tsagarakis, S. (2018). Microbiome and diabetes: Where are we now? *Diabetes Research and Clinical Practice, 146*, 111–118. https://doi.org/10.1016/j.diabres.2018.10.008

Venkataraman, A., Sieber, J. R., Schmidt, A. W., Waldron, C., Theis, K. R., & Schmidt, T. M. (2016). Variable responses of human microbiomes to dietary supplementation with resistant starch. *Microbiome, 4*(1). https://doi.org/10.1186/s40168-016-0178-x

Vigil, P., Meléndez, J., Petkovic, G., & Del Río, J. P. (2022). The importance of estradiol for body weight regulation in women. *Frontiers in Endocrinology, 13*, 951186. https://doi.org/10.3389/fendo.2022.951186

Wachsmuth, H. R., Weninger, S. N., & Duca, F. A. (2022). Role of the gut–brain axis in energy and glucose metabolism. *Experimental and Molecular Medicine, 54*(4), 377–392. https://doi.org/10.1038/s12276-021-00677-w

Wu, J., Wang, K., Wang, X., Pang, Y., & Jiang, C. (2020). The role of the gut microbiome and its metabolites in metabolic diseases. *Protein & Cell, 12*(5), 360–373. https://doi.org/10.1007/s13238-020-00814-7

Xiao, T., Wu, S., Cheng, Y., Zhao, C., Han Seung Jin, Yan, N., Xu, J., Wu, Y.-R., Li, C., Shao, Q., & Sheng, X. (2018). Butyrate upregulates the TLR4 expression and the phosphorylation of MAPKs and NK-κB in colon cancer cell in vitro. *Oncology Letters*. https://doi.org/10.3892/ol.2018.9201

Xu, M., Cen, M., Shen, Y., Zhu, Y., Cheng, F., Tang, L., Hu, W., & Dai, N. (2020). Deoxycholic acid-induced gut dysbiosis disrupts bile acid enterohepatic circulation and promotes intestinal inflammation. *Digestive Diseases and Sciences, 66*(2), 568–576. https://doi.org/10.1007/s10620-020-06208-3

Yang, Q., Liang, Q., Balakrishnan, B., Belobrajdic, D., Feng, Q.-J., & Zhang, W. (2020). Role of dietary nutrients in the modulation of gut microbiota: A narrative review. *Nutrients, 12*(2), 381. https://doi.org/10.3390/nu12020381

Yao, Y., Cai, X., Fei, W., Ye, Y., Zhao, M., & Zheng, C. (2020). The role of short-chain fatty acids in immunity, inflammation and metabolism. *Critical Reviews in Food Science and Nutrition, 62*(1), 1–12. https://doi.org/10.1080/10408398.2020.1854675

Zhang, B., Shen, S., Gu, T., Hong, T., Liu, J., Sun, J., Wang, H., Bi, Y., & Zhu, D.1 (2019). Increased circulating conjugated primary bile acids are associated with hyperandrogenism in women with polycystic ovary syndrome. Journal of Steroid Biochemistry and Molecular Biology, 189, 171–175. https://doi.org/10.1016/j.jsbmb.2019.03.005.

Zhang, W., An, Y., Qin, X., Wu, X., Wang, X., Hou, H., Song, X., Liu, T., Wang, B., Huang, X., & Cao, H. (2021). Gut microbiota-derived metabolites in colorectal cancer: The bad and the challenges. *Frontiers in Oncology, 11*. https://doi.org/10.3389/fonc.2021.739648

Zhao, L., Lou, H., Peng, Y., Chen, S., Zhang, Y., & Li, X. (2019). Comprehensive relationships between gut microbiome and faecal metabolome in individuals with type 2 diabetes and its complications. *Endocrine, 66*(3), 526–537. https://doi.org/10.1007/s12020-019-02103-8

Zhao, M., Chu, J., Feng, S., Guo, C., Xue, B., He, K., & Li, L. (2023). Immunological mechanisms of inflammatory diseases caused by gut microbiota dysbiosis: A review. *Biomedicine & Pharmacotherapy, 164*(1), 114985. https://doi.org/10.1016/j.biopha.2023.114985

Zivkovic, A. M., Telis, N., German, J. B., & Hammock, B. D. (2011). Dietary omega-3 fatty acids aid in the modulation of inflammation and metabolic health. *California Agriculture, 65*(3), 106–111. https://doi.org/10.3733/ca.v065n03p106

GPSR Compliance

The European Union's (EU) General Product Safety Regulation (GPSR) is a set of rules that requires consumer products to be safe and our obligations to ensure this.

If you have any concerns about our products, you can contact us on ProductSafety@springernature.com

In case Publisher is established outside the EU, the EU authorized representative is:

Springer Nature Customer Service Center GmbH
Europaplatz 3
69115 Heidelberg, Germany

Batch number: 10725825

Printed by Printforce, the Netherlands